Reverse Diabetes

12-WEEK CHALLENGE

PRAISE FOR REVERSE DIABETES

"This book is great. I learned a lot about good food choices and foods to avoid. It also contains great recipes for diabetics that are healthy and delicious. Would recommend this book to anyone with diabetes or prediabetes. The section on calories, sugar, and carbohydrates found in different foods was a big help in planning my everyday meals. The exercise section was also very helpful. Already lost 15 pounds." —**J.S. MD**

"This book answered so many questions when I was newly diagnosed with diabetes. It's a long-term book for living with and reversing diabetes in addition to being very encouraging and upbeat. The organization of the book and the layout are reader friendly. I have marked it liberally with a highlighter and refer to it several times a week."
—Elizabeth Allanson

"This is a WONDERFUL book, it is easy to read and understand on any level. No big scientific words… Just regular words and pictures :-) It takes you step by step on HOW to improve your life with diabetes and how to minimize the symptoms and reverse diabetes. GREAT BOOK!" —**S. McGee**

"Love this book and it has really helped me. Very well thought out with clear explanations. Worth getting and I will be recommending it!"—**A'anna T. Williams**

"I found this book educational. I like the clear descriptions as well as the variety of menus… I will go back to it often." —**Gisela M. Damandl**

"I love this book. I am not diabetic; however, I did want to shed unwanted pounds. This book teaches how to keep your sugar steady so you aren't constantly hungry. An easy read!" —**Shakala**

"Excellent book to read if you are diabetic. Many helpful suggestions were presented. Often it just takes a few lifestyle tweaks to make diabetes management possible."
—Karen L. Pitts

"My husband found out he had type 2 diabetes and I knew nothing about it or how to cook and care for him. This book was excellent. The price and packaging were great as well. Recommended purchase." —**Mamad**

"This is great, explains everything so well… This is a great start to YOU helping yourself fight and get rid of diabetes for good. No need for medications, that's what you are working for!" —**Nancy J.**

Revised & Updated!

Reader's Digest

Reverse Diabetes

12-WEEK CHALLENGE

Gain Energy Lose Inches!

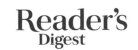

Reader's Digest

New York, NY / Montreal

ISBN 978-1-62145-851-7 (paperback)
ISBN 978-1-62145-853-1 (e-pub)

Printed in China
10 9 8 7 6 5 4 3 2 1

Note to Readers

The information in this book should not be substituted for, or used to alter, medical therapy without your doctor's advice. For a specific health problem, consult your physician for guidance. The mention of any products, retail businesses, or websites in this book does not imply or constitute an endorsement by Trusted Media Brands, Inc.

Credits

PAGES 192–193: "International Table of Glycemic Index and Glycemic Load Values 2002," Kaye Foster-Powell, Susanna H. A. Holt, and Janette C. Brand-Miller, *American Journal of Clinical Nutrition*, vol. 76, no. 1 (2002), 5–56. Additional data from www.glycemicindex.com, www. mypyramid.gov, and www.ars.usda.gov.

PHOTOS:
Getty Images: *front cover left* Damir Khabirov; *front cover right* Science Photo Library; *42 (16)* Brian Hagiwara; *43 (17), 127* Image Source; *80* Jose Luis Pelaez, Inc.; *95* IT Stock; *105* PeopleImages; *136* Jupiterimages

Shutterstock: *10, 75, 90, 102, 116, 119, 122, 129, 135* Monkey Business Images; *16, 19, 77, 142* Prostock-studio; *24* Inside Creative House; *26* Josep Suria; *28* New Africa; *31, back cover right* JLco Julia Amaral; *33* Rawpixel.com; *38* Ahmet Misirligul; *40 (1)* Tim UR; *40 (2)* Irina Gutyryak; *40 (3)* AmyLv; *40 (4)* Happy Author; *40 (5)* Misses Jones; *41 (6)* Anthony Hersey; *41 (7)* Nik Merkulov; *41 (8)* Elena Zajchikova; *41 (9)* Bartas Artiom; *41 (10)* Suradech Prapairat; *41 (11)* pukao; *42 (12)* Pun foto; *42 (13)* Andrey_Kuzmin; *42 (14)* draconus; *42 (15)* Africa Studio; *43 (18)* baibaz; *43 (19)* MaraZe; *43 (20)* Maria Kovalets; *47* Nataliia Sirobaba; *49* etorres; *51* Nata Bene; *53* Asya Nurullina; *76* chomplearn; *85* Shoaib_Mughal; *86, 125, back cover left,* Rido; *88* Jacob Lund; *93* MaeManee; *98* Kostiantyn Voitenko; *101, 169 left* PeopleImages.com - Yuri A; *103* studioloco; *124* fizkes; *126* Ljupco Smokovski; *145* mimagephotography; *147-169* popicon; *147* luckyraccoon; *151* Syda Productions; *153* pics five; *157* Halfpoint; *163* Photoroyalty; *170* DC Studio; *173* Kostikova Natalia

All other images copyright Trusted Media Brands, Inc.

DI · A · BE · TES

(noun): a disorder of carbohydrate metabolism characterized by inadequate production or usage of insulin and causing excessive levels of glucose in the blood and urine

RE · VERSE

(verb): to turn in the opposite direction or send on the opposite course

Contents

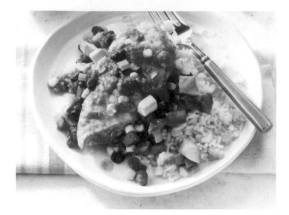

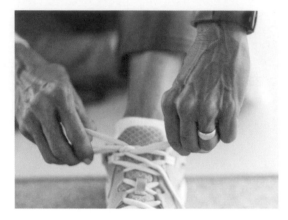

PART ONE

EAT
to Reverse Diabetes

PART TWO

MOVE
to Reverse Diabetes

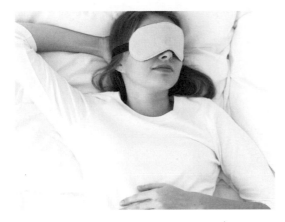

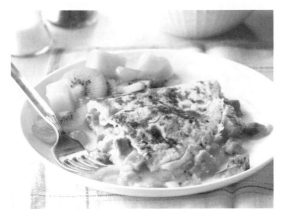

Diabetes Is No Longer Something to Fear

UNLIKE SEVERAL DECADES AGO, diabetes is a diagnosis that comes with plenty of tools to manage it. Personally, as someone with a family history of type 2 diabetes, I've seen firsthand this evolution from a feeling of apprehension to now one of determination and possibilities. Professionally, as a registered dietitian nutritionist (RDN), chef, and cookbook author, I've tried my best to be at least one small part of that solution—writing three diabetes cookbooks to date.

Today, you can feel comforted in knowing that managing your diabetes is not something you need to do all on your own. Many people, organizations, and publications offer tremendous care, support, and reliable, evidence-based information. Think of it as a team approach with this book, *Reverse Diabetes: 12-Week Challenge*, as an integral part of your support team.

Being up to date is key. The prevention and treatment of diabetes has changed over the years—including in the 13 years since this book was originally published. This completely revised edition—based on the latest research about what works—showcases how restrictive diets, avoidance, and a one-size-fits-all approach are no

longer the focus. Rather, individualization and "What can I eat?" rather than "What can't I eat?" are guiding principles. Strict counting and precise calculations are not necessary. A variety of colorful vegetables, whole grains, beans, nuts, seeds, and yes, even fruits, are celebrated. And even that slice of birthday cake can fit into a plan for type 2 diabetes. You'll use the Plate Approach to effortlessly put your personalized diabetes eating plan into practice.

Making smart choices is the aim. Carbs, including sugars, are not the enemy; but choosing mostly nutrient-rich sources of carbohydrates and balancing them throughout the day is key. Healthy fats and protein are beneficial. The concept of "skinny" or drastic weight loss is out. And aiming to lose 10 percent of your body weight (not what a chart or social media says) is the research-backed approach. Step by step, *Reverse Diabetes* shows you how to achieve these eating and healthy weight goals—and more.

How does this book do that? It starts with a comprehensive, yet "can do" attitude and a simple, user-friendly style, focusing on three areas where you can be the boss of your disease—eat, move, and choose. It takes an overall lifestyle approach to managing your blood glucose and A1C levels, and diabetes in general.

The plan features clear and doable goals for each of these three areas. It offers more than 60 tasty diabetes-friendly recipes, sample meal plans, easy-to-implement exercise strategies, and lots of friendly yet impactful diabetes-focused lifestyle advice, such as walking five days a week and getting restful sleep. The nutrition information offered throughout the book is based on current research and facts, not fads. And it can be adapted to your preferences and needs—for instance, if you choose to adopt a plant-forward diet, travel frequently and need to dine out often, or work a night shift, you can still easily follow the 12-Week Reverse Diabetes Challenge.

Plus, the book includes numerous interactive quizzes, checklists, trackers, and other tools to help you easily transform the book's guidance into action. You'll find everything you need to follow the 12-Week Challenge within the pages of this book, but if you prefer to go digital, you can do that, too, with the online tools at thehealthy.com /reversediabetes.

Finally, it's important to know that what you do today to manage diabetes will change over time. Beyond the 12-Week Challenge, and throughout the weeks, months, and years to come, the knowledge and tools you'll find in this book will help guide you in continuously evaluating and adjusting your approach to diabetes management.

While diabetes is a serious medical condition, take heart in knowing that it is fully manageable. You—along with your team—can help determine your healthy future and put your diabetes into remission. You'll be so thankful you chose this book to help you do just that.

Cheers to your good health!
JACKIE NEWGENT, RDN, CDN

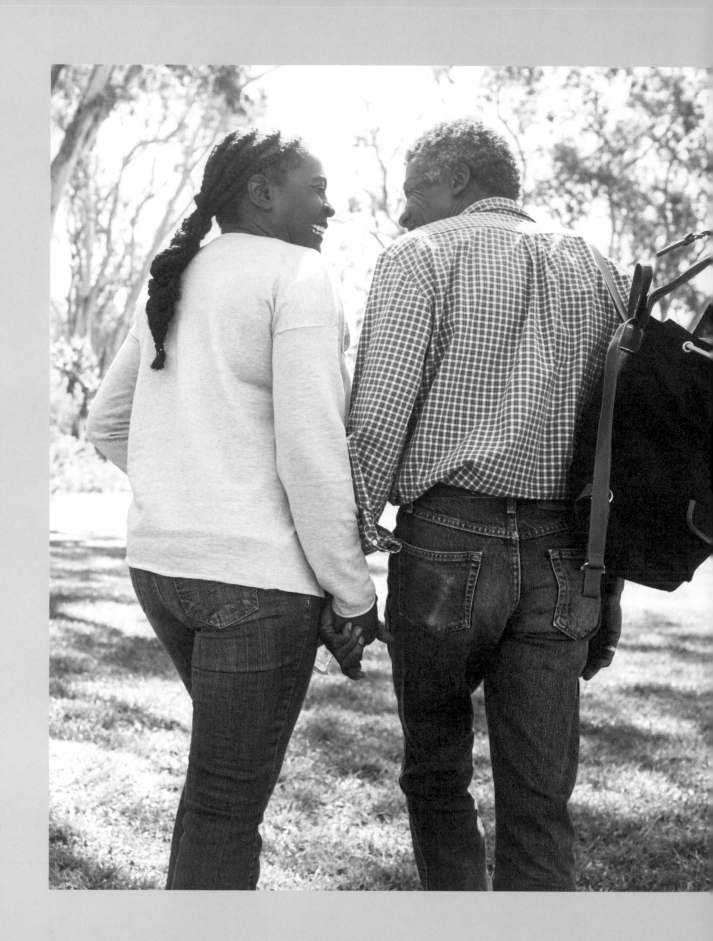

Introducing the Eat, Move, Choose Plan

Can you really reverse type 2 diabetes? Absolutely! Ground-breaking studies on real patients have shown that it's possible to send the disease into complete remission—to erase all signs of it within a year. This turnaround is possible no matter how long you've had diabetes.

Doctors accomplished this through weight-loss surgery on obese people, but even without surgery, it's now clear that *you* have the power to reverse the course of your disease—to turn back the clock on insulin resistance, the metabolic problem at the core of the condition, and see better blood sugar levels again, along with vastly improved overall health. All with far less hassle than you might think.

A wave of research shows that by making easy, manageable changes to your daily habits you can achieve remarkable improvements in your A1C level (an indirect measure of your blood glucose levels over the last three months), your weight, and other health markers. If you take diabetes medications or use insulin, you may be able to reduce your dose or even tear up your prescription, depending on where you are in the course of your disease.

Even modest lifestyle changes can have profound benefits. For instance, simply taking a brisk walk three times a week can significantly lower blood sugar. Eating a bit less every day, but *not* dramatically cutting calories, can lead to long-term weight loss, a vital goal for most people with type 2 diabetes. Swapping certain foods for healthier choices can not only improve your body's sensitivity to the hormone insulin—essentially reversing the course of your diabetes—but can also keep a lid on your risk for heart disease, without punishing your palate. Scientists have even discovered that reining in stress can lower blood sugar and decrease the amount of harmful fat, known as visceral fat, that you carry deep in your belly, fat that makes blood sugar management more difficult.

Reverse Diabetes incorporates all the newest findings about the best ways to thrive with this condition and translates these revelations into a 12-week challenge with simple, clear goals and easy-to-follow advice. But first, a bit more about the new cutting-edge science upon which this book is based.

The New Thinking on Reversing Diabetes

THERE'S ONE WORD that medical researchers rarely utter—and it's this: Cure.

Yet, during a presentation at a science conference, that's exactly the word researchers from the Diabetes Remission Clinical Trial (DiRECT) used to describe the outlook for people with type 2 diabetes. This ongoing study of hundreds of people with diabetes has revealed a powerful cocktail of lifestyle approaches can help drive diabetes into complete remission. That means blood sugar remains in the healthy range, without the use of medication, month after month after month.

To help you achieve this enviable result, *Reverse Diabetes* addresses three key areas: eat, move, and choose. Let's take a closer look at how all three work together to help you put diabetes in your rear view mirror

The Reverse Diabetes Eat Plan: Smarter Carbs and Fat, More Protein and Veggies

The old thinking about diabetes and diet could be summed up in two words: Avoid sugar. That seemed logical; if diabetes causes high blood sugar,

why would you want to add to the problem by gobbling chocolate bars and guzzling liquid calories?

But sugar is just one ingredient in the nutritional pie. While it's still great to eat less of it, other dietary tweaks are proving just as powerful or even more so when it comes to managing and reversing diabetes.

The new advice:

Quit focusing on subtraction—because it usually backfires. If you've ever sworn off sugar or desserts, then you know this all too well. You might manage a few zero consumption days. Eventually, however, your cravings overpower your willpower, leading to more sweets than ever before.

Thankfully, there's a better way.

Instead of banning foods, think about adding nourishing foods that help maintain steady blood sugar levels and simultaneously lower your risk for heart disease.

On the Reverse Diabetes plan, you'll fill your plate with:

Produce. Consuming more fruit and non-starchy vegetables—nature's all-purpose disease fighters—appears to combat diabetes. People who eat three servings of fruit per day cut the risk for developing type 2 diabetes by 18 percent, finds research. On top of that, every serving of leafy green vegetables you consume per day—such as lettuce, spinach, broccoli, and others—may lower risk by another 9 percent.

How do fruits and veggies help? First, these healthy foods tend to be low in calories, which can help you lose fat. Second, fruits and vegetables tend to be rich in fiber, which helps to slow digestion, providing slow and even rises in blood sugar as well as curbing your appetite.

Finally, produce comes packed with healing nutrients such as antioxidants, vitamins, and minerals which are thought to help ease the insulin resistance that drives diabetes.

Smart proteins. Whether it comes from animals (poultry, seafood and beef) or plants (beans, soy, and nuts), protein helps to dampen appetite, making fat loss easier. It also doesn't affect blood sugar levels as much as carbohydrate-rich foods.

That said, not all protein-rich foods offer the same benefits.

Highly processed and fatty meats have been linked to an increased risk of diabetes, whereas leaner, minimally processed options such as chicken breast, seafood, beans, and low-fat Greek or Skyr yogurt help to lower your risk. In the Reverse Diabetes 12-week challenge, you'll learn how to shift your protein choices toward smart proteins that help you fill up on fewer calories.

Smart carbs. Minimally processed whole foods can be your best friends. Rich in digestion-slowing fiber and plant nutrients, these foods closely resemble their "right off the vine" state. Think sweet potatoes, brown rice, beans and lentils (which are also protein rich), and corn, among many other foods. In contrast, highly processed carbs such as white bread and sugar-sweetened foods digest quickly, sending blood sugar soaring.

Smart fats. Nuts, avocados, and olive oil are all top sources of monounsaturated fat. Unlike artery-clogging saturated fat (found in full-fat dairy and in meats) and trans fat (the fat in many snacks and fast foods), "monos" appear to fight heart disease. Even better, replacing "bad" fats with the mono-unsaturated variety combats insulin resistance, which we've already described as the key metabolic problem at the core of type 2 diabetes.

A high-mono diet can help people with type 2 diabetes control their A1C and weight, according to a study at the University of Cincinnati. The study's lead author, nutritionist Bonnie Brehm, PhD, says the key to successfully re-crafting your diet is "to start with small, achievable goals"—which is exactly what you'll be doing during your 12-week challenge.

Don't focus on forbidden foods. Instead, think about adding to your diet foods that help maintain steady blood sugar levels.

The Reverse Diabetes Move Plan: Revving Your Metabolic Engine

Play a few sets of pickleball. Take a long hike. Spend an afternoon planting perennials. What do these enjoyable activities have in common? As in all forms of exercise, they burn up blood sugar as well as reduce insulin resistance, making cells more sensitive to the hormone and thereby putting your disease into reverse.

Here's how it works. Normally, in people who don't have diabetes, insulin easily unlocks muscle cells so they let in glucose (blood sugar) from the bloodstream to use as fuel. But if you have type 2 diabetes, your body has become less responsive to insulin, and your cells remain "locked up" to glucose, leaving it to build up in the blood. That can cause damage to tiny blood vessels and nerves. Over time, chronically elevated blood sugar can lead to a long list of diabetes complications: vision loss, serious skin ulcers, kidney disease, and others.

Exercise encourages the body to become more sensitive to insulin. Hardworking muscle cells that desperately need glucose will go to extreme measures to get it, producing chemicals that lower their resistance to the hormone.

That's not all. Reams of studies show that regular exercise can help improve hemoglobin A1C levels, lower triglycerides and cholesterol, and slow the development of diabetes-related complications such as peripheral neuropathy, the nerve damage that can lead to numbness and pain.

You may be wondering how hard and long you need to work out to see results.

The answer: A lot less than you probably think.

The results of the The Look AHEAD (Action for Health in Diabetes) trial (one of the largest randomized trials evaluating physical activity and

No Drastic Measures Needed

It's so easy to get caught up in trends, especially when headlines scream that high-intensity interval training (HIIT) is the BEST exercise for people with diabetes. Or that extreme low carb diets or intermittent fasting help to speed weight loss.

First, based on the DIETFITS (Diet Intervention Examining the Factors Interacting with Treatment Success) study, many eating approaches can help people lose weight and lower blood sugar and cholesterol. Though study participants might lose more on one type of diet initially, participants tend to end up in the same place long term.

Because of that, researchers from a range of institutions have concluded: Most diets—ranging from low carb to low fat to intermittent fasting—can lead to weight loss and healthy outcomes, as long as people follow them consistently.

Almost no one can consistently cut all carbs from their diet or only eat every other day.

That's because these types of diets literally go against human nature—and might even be dangerous (by causing fluctuations in blood sugar or causing deficiencies in some nutrients).

Rather than force yourself to do the most extreme diet or most intense exercise regimen, embrace changes that feel like a good fit, that you can maintain, and that you think you might even come to enjoy. The 12-week challenge will show you how.

diabetes) are in and they're promising. People who moved for 175 minutes a week improved a host of factors—weight loss, blood sugar control, reduced blood pressure and cholesterol–than people who didn't exercise. That's just 20-25 minutes a day.

And it doesn't have to be done all at once.

Sprinkling activity throughout your day—especially short walks after meals—helps to blunt

Drop a Little, Reverse A Lot

By now, you've no doubt heard about the dangers of abdominal fat.

Excess body fat triggers inflammation that can raise your risk of a range of health problems, including heart disease. Here's more: Excess fat within and around your liver can boost glucose production, making your A1C numbers jump. In the pancreas, excess fat hinders the function of beta cells, which make insulin.

This new understanding of how abdominal fat interacts with blood sugar means that physicians now see weight management as one of the most important pillars of diabetes treatment and prevention. "Treating obesity is treating the core of the problem," says Osama Hamdy, MD, of the Joslin Diabetes Center in Boston.

The great news: It only takes a small amount of fat loss to turn blood sugar problems around.

According to the DiRECT trial mentioned earlier, dropping roughly 22 pounds (10 kilograms) is enough to drive diabetes into complete remission for many people. According to other research, smaller changes of the scale—as little as a couple pounds—can dramatically help you improve blood sugar levels, especially when you incorporate other lifestyle factors (such as diet, exercise, mood, and sleep).

On the Reverse Diabetes plan, you'll address excess body fat in three ways.

1. Through walking and strength training, you'll increase how many calories you burn each day.
2. By using our handy plate method coupled with research-supported mindfulness techniques, you'll automatically consume the right portions for fat loss—no calorie counting required.
3. By addressing your mindset—and specifically sleep—you'll unlock more energy (which makes exercise so much easier). Your appetite and cravings will also drop, making it easier for you to follow your Eat goals.

the post meal rise in blood glucose, insulin, and triglycerides, finds research. You might start with one 5-to 15-minute walk after lunch or dinner. Over the 12-week challenge, you'll progress to up to 45 minutes per session.

Want to lower your blood sugar even more? Most experts agree that adding strength training to your routine is essential, too. Resistance training builds muscle, which helps to improve blood sugar control and decreases insulin resistance.

On the Reverse Diabetes plan, you'll combine both forms of exercise, starting at a duration and pace that works for your lifestyle and fitness level.

The Reverse Diabetes Choose Plan: Stress Poses a Triple Whammy When You Have Diabetes

For starters, it leads to unhealthy habits. You know the usual suspects: eating junk food, skipping exercise, drinking too much alcohol. You also may forget to take your medications or just decide you can't be bothered with them.

On top of that, stress raises blood sugar even in the absence of unhealthy behaviors. When you're stressed, your body produces more of the "stress hormone" cortisol. Cortisol helps to mobilize your "fight or flight" response in the event of a crisis—a fire, for instance. But it also raises blood sugar. That means that over the long-term, chronic stress can pose a serious problem. "High levels of stress hormones can put your diabetes out of control," says Wayne Katon, MD, University of Washington professor of psychiatry.

Finally, over time, stress can also increase the amount of fat you accumulate around your internal organs. This type of fat produces dangerous chemicals that damage the arteries and increase the risk for heart attacks.

Just reading about all of that is pretty stressful! Thankfully, you have the power to manage stress. The Reverse Diabetes Choose Plan will show you how.

By inspiring yourself daily, you'll stay fired up and motivated to eat well, move, and practice other healthy behaviors, regardless of the curveballs life tosses your way. And by improving sleep and practicing self care, you'll boost your stress resilience, which means you'll more easily weather life storms.

End result: Your blood sugar will improve. In one study, people with type 2 diabetes who learned to de-stress by meditating (which is just one of the tools you'll learn in the Choose plan) dropped their A1C scores by a nifty 0.48 percent, on average. Big bonus: Their blood pressure fell, too, by six points.

Why Sleep Matters

Here's a piece of news that you should take lying down: Getting a better night's rest can significantly lower your blood sugar and help you reverse your diabetes. A University of Chicago study found that type 2 diabetes patients who get by on just five hours a night may be able to lower their A1C numbers by more than 1 percent by stretching their nightly slumber to eight hours. Meanwhile a review showed that sleep quality and timing also impacts blood sugar levels.

Why is sleep so important when you have diabetes? No one is sure, but a few facts are clear. Studies show that sleep deprivation triggers insulin resistance. It also causes hormones that turn down your appetite to plummet. At the same time, other hormones that make you hungry—especially for carbohydrates—shift into high gear. That's a setup for weight gain, which makes insulin resistance even worse.

Getting a better night's rest can significantly lower your blood sugar.

Eat, Move, and Choose to Reverse Diabetes

BY LOSING WEIGHT and lowering your blood sugar and your resistance to insulin, you can put your disease in reverse. That simple, stunning fact was the inspiration behind *Reverse Diabetes* and the Eat, Move, Choose Plan. This unique program, based on the best new science, is designed to help you—step by step and day by day—make the small changes in your life that will add up to better health, along with greater energy, a slimmer silhouette, and happier moods. The time to start it? Today. In fact, you can start right this second if you wish by putting down this book and going for a walk or eating a carrot. Yes, it's that easy!

A Comprehensive Three-Part Plan

Dealing with diabetes can feel overwhelming at times. But bringing the disease under control is an important task, and there's no one better qualified to do it than you. (Doctors can prescribe medicines if you need them, but they can't cure or even manage the disease for you.) If you take the right steps, you can live a full and active life and even feel healthier than you have in years. We've charted the path for you with the Eat, Move, Choose Plan. It leaves nothing to chance—and if you follow it closely, we guarantee you'll see improvements in your blood sugar readings and probably your cholesterol profile, too.

In each of the three parts of the plan, we've spelled out crystal-clear goals along with the concrete steps you'll take to achieve them. On the Eat plan you'll discover surprising truths about what you should and shouldn't pile onto your plate when you have diabetes. For instance, consuming more fruits and vegetables is more important than ever, while the message about carbs and fats has changed considerably over the years. It's no longer about finding the willpower to eliminate sugar, junk foods, and other highly processed fare. Rather, you'll learn how to fill up on wholesome smart carbs and smart fats that help to automatically eat less of the other stuff. You'll also keep blood sugar on an even keel and turn down cravings.

Portion control is also key, of course, and we've found a way to make it truly easy—no calorie counting required.

17

One of the most effective ways to reverse insulin resistance is to get off the couch and move your body. You may not think of yourself as the exercise type, but don't write off this critical portion of the plan. You'll start the Move plan with as much walking you can comfortably handle, whether that's 2 minutes or 25. We'll also help you build up your muscle mass right at home, no equipment required, with a strengthening program we call the Sugar Buster Routine. Again, you can do it in just minutes a day, and it has no fitness prerequisite. On the Move plan we'll also encourage you to sneak more everyday exercise into your life by spending some time yanking weeds in the garden, washing the car by hand, or simply taking the stairs instead of the elevator. These small choices may not seem like much, but the cumulative effect is much greater than you might think.

Getting enough sleep, finding ways to combat stress, and keeping your motivation soaring are all vitally important aspects of good diabetes management, and they're all part of the Choose plan, too.

Tracking Your Progress

Reversing diabetes isn't something that happens overnight (although getting a good night's sleep really does help keep blood sugar levels in check!). It's something you do every day—starting today. Throughout the book, you'll find a number of tools that will make planning, tracking, shopping, and preparing food easier than ever. Feel free to copy and print them. Or, if you prefer to go higher tech, you can find these tools online at thehealthy.com/reversediabetes.

Scan to find the tools online.

Like a personal trainer, motivational life coach, and nutritional consultant rolled into one, the 12-Week Challenge will suggest weekly goals. Each week builds on the one that came before. You'll start slowly—with fitness, sleep, stress management, and nutritional goals you can handle. As the weeks progress, you'll take on a little more. By the end, you'll be a pro at the Reverse Diabetes lifestyle. Even better, your health will have transformed—and you'll look and feel absolutely amazing.

At the beginning of each week, we recommend you use our handy meal planning template to plan your meals for the next seven days (see page 176). This is a powerful and important strategy for keeping you on top of your Eat goals. Use the more than 60 diabetes-friendly recipes in the Recipes section to help you. Knowing what you'll eat during the week translates into knowing exactly what you'll buy at the supermarket. That means you'll come home with shopping bags full of smart, delicious, healthy foods for weight loss and better blood sugar control—instead of foods full of empty calories that are so easy to buy on a whim at the grocery store.

By tracking your progress over 12 weeks of the challenge, you'll notice and celebrate every success, discover areas that need improvement, feel inspired to get up and do it all again

Complications Are Not Inevitable

It was once thought that just about everyone with diabetes would eventually develop complications of the disease, such as nerve damage, foot problems, and vision problems. That's simply not true. By keeping your blood sugar in the normal range, you can slash your risk of these health problems and live a healthy life like anyone else.

tomorrow, and build motivation to get back on track if you've had a setback. You'll learn new things about yourself and your body—such as how daily stress reduction and exercise influence your blood sugar, how a few minutes of advance planning makes grabbing a healthy snack a snap, and how a week or a month of healthy choices pays off in lower numbers on the bathroom scale, on the tape measure you wrap around your middle, and on your blood sugar meter.

We recommend spending a few moments on Sunday evening to look back at the previous week (and ahead to your goals for the coming week). Mull over how you did against the goals on the Eat, Move, Choose Plan. Be sure to give yourself a nice pat on the back for anything and everything you've worked so hard to achieve, whether it was eating more vegetables, adding five minutes to your walks, or trying out one of our instant stress-buster strategies. Also note instances when you slipped up. Think about what got you off track and what you'd do differently the next time.

Why the Plan Works

Lots of plans offer good ideas about what *should* work when it comes to weight loss and diabetes management. Here's what makes the Eat, Move, Choose Plan so uniquely effective.

It doesn't rely on calorie-cutting. This plan corrects fundamental errors that people make while trying to lose weight, such as skipping breakfast, attempting to cut too much fat from their diets, and going overboard on starchy foods. Another common mistake: trying to lose weight by obsessing about calories. Our Reverse Diabetes Plate will show you how to eat balanced portions of smart carbs, smart proteins, and smart fats—all automatically portioned for weight loss, no calorie counting required.

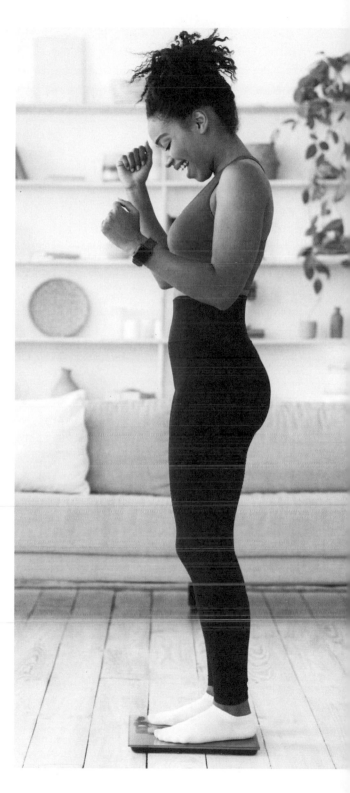

You can eat foods you like. This plan never restricts *what* you can eat, although you may need to eat favorite foods less often, in smaller portions, or prepared in different ways. It won't feel like a diet, just a healthier way of eating.

It's a plan you can live with. Doctors and dietitians find that many people have an extremely tough time staying on diets that are radically low in either carbohydrates or fat. People give up on these diets because they're just too restrictive. This is a plan you can live with for life.

It's gradual. We won't ask you to change your life overnight. You can incorporate the steps in the Eat and Choose plans as quickly or as slowly as you wish. And the Move plan was designed to start you off slowly and gradually build you up to doing more exercise as you get fitter and fitter.

It's easy to follow, at home and away from home. There's no calorie or carbohydrate counting, you don't have to try to make sense of the confusing glycemic index, and we won't ask you to eat your burger without a bun or pass up potatoes. You're allowed to eat bread and pasta, and even dessert, in reasonable amounts. Yes, you will need to make some changes—for instance, fill your plate with more non-starchy vegetables, eat fewer french fries and potatoes, cut back a bit on portion sizes overall, and get off the couch for some exercise almost every day—but they aren't big ones. And we know you're ready for change, or you wouldn't be reading this book.

Our Promise

By the end of 12 weeks on the Eat, Move, Choose Plan, you'll be well on your way to losing 10 percent of your body weight—a goal that in one major study, the Diabetes Obesity Intervention Trial (DO IT), led to a significant drop in fasting blood sugar levels and to a reduction in medication use for many study volunteers. You will also have reaped a number of other important health benefits. Our promise to you:

Weight loss that works. We'll never ask you to follow a gimmicky diet, eat special "diabetic" foods, to weigh or measure every morsel, deprive yourself of your favorite edibles, or sign up for a boot-camp-level exercise routine. Radical overhauls may produce short-term results but can't stand up to the test of real-world living. That's the beauty and the power of the Eat, Move, Choose Plan. You'll follow clear, simple steps to success that are proven to work no matter what daily living has in store for you. We'll show you which changes have the most impact and how to fit them into your life. For example, you'll learn how to use your dinner plate to eat perfectly sized portions, how to fit walking and strength-training exercises into the busiest days, and how to get more sleep for automatic weight loss and effortless blood sugar benefits.

Introducing the Reverse Diabetes Toolbox

Throughout this book, you'll find several powerful tools that will make reversing diabetes a whole lot easier. These include:

- **A meal planner** that will help you figure out what you're making for the week ahead
- A **shopping list** and **grocery checklist** that helps you get what you need at the store, without forgetting any essentials
- An optional **food diary,** to get a baseline read on your eating habits

Scan to find the tools online.

Less abdominal fat. The Eat, Move, Choose Plan uses a one-two-three strategy (the right foods and exercise, plus lifestyle tweaks including stress reduction) to trim belly fat—something that losing weight by simply cutting calories cannot accomplish. All weight loss is good, but it's especially important to get rid of fat deep in your abdomen—the stuff that wraps around internal organs, pumping blood sugar-raising compounds into your bloodstream around the clock. This plan shrinks it.

Better blood sugar management. Losing a fairly modest amount of weight can lower your blood sugar by a whopping 25 percent, enough to let some people reduce the dosage of their diabetes medications or stop them entirely. In the DO IT study, people who shed 10 percent of their body weight (that's 17 pounds if you weigh 170) saw their fasting blood glucose levels fall from an average of 170 mg/dl—well into dangerously elevated territory—to 125 mg/dl, a level considered pre-diabetic. They also lowered their A1C levels from an average of 8 (normal for people with diabetes, but considered a risk for diabetes complications), to 6.7—below the 7 target recommended by the American Diabetes Association.

Improved insulin sensitivity. People with type 2 diabetes are insulin resistant. Exercise, trimming deep belly fat, reducing stress, and eating a healthy diet—all of which you'll do on the Eat, Move, Choose Plan—work together to restore insulin sensitivity. In the DO IT study, sensitivity improved by two- to five-fold—enough that 18 of 25 study volunteers who took diabetes medications were able to stop.

Protection from diabetes complications. By following the research-tested strategies in this book, you will lower your blood pressure, reduce heart-threatening LDL cholesterol and triglycerides, and raise heart-protecting HDL cholesterol. The Eat, Move, Choose Plan also helps cool chronic inflammation, a potent risk factor for heart disease. The result: powerful protection against heart attacks, strokes, congestive heart failure, and other forms of cardiovascular disease.

But that's not all. Lowering your blood sugar will also protect you from major diabetes complications including vision loss due to diabetic retinopathy, kidney failure, and amputation due to nerve damage and poor circulation.

Involving Your Doctor and Dietitian

To get the most out of the Eat, Move, Choose Plan, it's important for you to talk with your health care provider and with a registered dietitian or certified diabetes educator before you begin. These members of your diabetes care team can help you adjust and adapt the elements of the plan to your unique needs. They will assess your readiness for exercise, and recommend a blood sugar testing strategy that will help you avoid highs and lows and a medication strategy that will keep your blood sugar within a healthy range. Here's what your conversation should cover.

The best exercise for you. Most people with diabetes will be able to start the gentle, progressive Move plan just as it is. But if you take insulin or oral diabetes drugs called insulin secretagogues, you will need to discuss how to time exercise, medication doses, and perhaps a carbohydrate-rich snack so that exercise doesn't lead to dangerously low blood sugar.

If you've already experienced diabetes complications, your doctor may recommend adjusting your exercise routine. For example, if you have nerve damage called peripheral neuropathy, your health care provider may recommend activities such as swimming, biking, or arm exercises instead of walking to avoid damage to your feet that could lead to infection. Your health-care provider may also recommend heart tests, such as an exercise stress test, before giving you the green light to exercise.

Meal adjustments. If you use carbohydrate counting to help control blood sugar, a dietitian can help you fit that eating strategy into the Eat guidelines. Your doctor, certified diabetes educator, or registered dietitian can also help you customize the Eat portion of the Eat, Move, Choose Plan so that the calories and food choices fit your needs.

A blood sugar testing schedule. Your diabetes management team can help you decide how often to perform blood sugar checks as you embark on the plan. Regular checks will show you how changes in your food choices, exercise level, stress, and sleep alter your blood sugar and will help your doctor decide whether you can reduce medication dosages. (Never alter your dosage or stop taking a drug on your own.)

A checkup plan. Expect your blood sugar to become easier to control and to move closer to a normal range as you progress through the 12-week Eat, Move, Choose Plan. If you're using medication, ask your doctor how often you should check in or make appointments to reassess your dosages and prescriptions. You may need to change one or both as your body becomes more sensitive to insulin.

You Are Not Alone

Wherever you are on your diabetes journey—whether you have just been diagnosed, have been grappling with the disease for years, or even just want to drop a few pounds and get your blood glucose on a more even keel—know that many

Can You Get Off Your Meds?

For some people on the Eat, Move, Choose Plan, one of the biggest payoffs will be taking less diabetes medication or even getting off diabetes medication altogether. We can't make promises. You need to make treatment decisions with your doctor, especially when it comes to any changes in medication. And diabetes is a progressive disease—the longer you have it, the more likely you'll need pharmaceutical help to manage it. But here's what you might be able to expect if you succeed in bringing your blood sugar down to the following levels:

126 to 140 or 150 mg/dl: While still above normal, these levels are low enough that you might be able to reduce your dosage.

150 to 200 mg/dl: The chances are good that continuing to follow the plan may allow you to get off medication. For now, however, you may still need medication and perhaps occasional doses of insulin.

Above 200 mg/dl: You may need medication or full-time insulin coverage, and possibly both, but the plan may let you reduce your doses or make other adjustments. What's more, it will most likely lower your blood pressure and improve your cholesterol numbers. And of course, you'll enjoy a greater sense of control over your health.

readers just like you have used the advice in this book to improve their symptoms and live longer and better. We here at The Healthy (a Reader's Digest brand) and Reader's Digest are cheering for you as you do the same. We'd love to hear about your diabetes journey at thehealthy.com/reversediabetes/shareyourstory.

Scan to share your story online.

Personal Contract

Keep this contract as a reminder of your commitment to the Eat, Move, Choose Plan and reversing your diabetes.

I vow that over the next 12 weeks I will learn and follow the steps to better blood sugar management and weight loss in the Eat, Move, Choose Plan.

Scan to find the contract online.

MY GOALS

My weight loss goal over the next 12 weeks (up to one pound a week is an appropriate target for most people): _____

My blood sugar goals over the next 12 weeks (discuss what goal is reasonable for you with your doctor or certified diabetes educator):

Fasting glucose: _____

A1C: _____

MY STRATEGIES

To reach these goals, I agree to:

1. Adopt the plan's strategies for getting more vegetables, fruit, whole grains, lean protein, low-fat dairy products, and good fats into my diet and for cutting back on saturated fat, trans fat, and refined carbohydrates.

2. Follow the Plate Approach at every meal to control portion sizes and calories.

3. Walk most days of the week and build up to performing the Sugar Buster Routine twice a week.

4. Make a good night's sleep a priority.

5. Practice a self-care technique every day.

6. Track my progress using the Reverse Diabetes tools.

7. Plan my meals in advance using the Reverse Diabetes tools.

8. Note my successes as well as my failures at the end of each week; I promise to cheer myself on every step of the way.

MY MOTIVATION

Here's why I want to do all I can to manage my diabetes:

1. _____

_____

_____

_____

2. _____

_____

_____

_____

3. _____

_____

_____

_____

Signed:_____

Date:_____

Witness (optional):_____

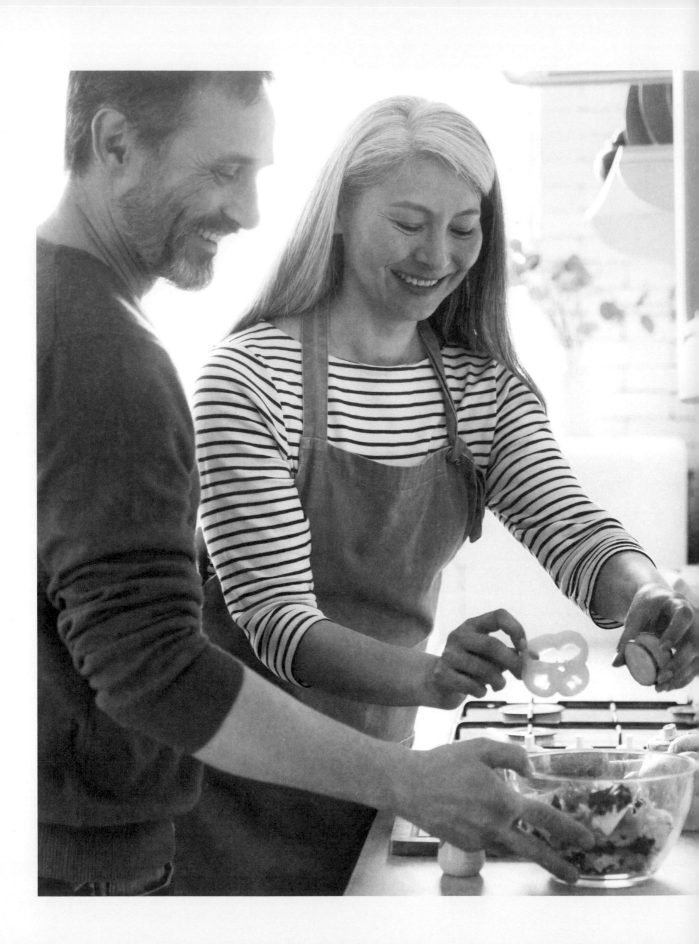

1

EAT
to Reverse Diabetes

- Delicious Foods
- Satisfying Meals
- Perfect Portions

The Plan

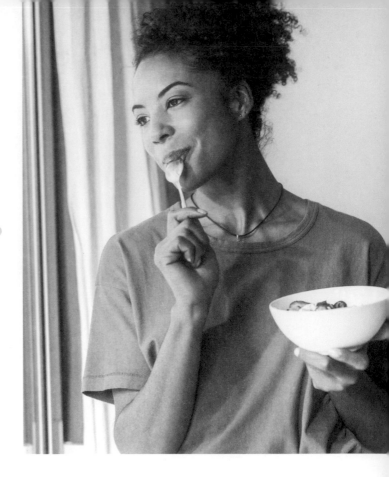

Eating to beat diabetes can seem awfully complicated and, well, intimidating. We've solved that problem by boiling down the best research-backed eating advice for people with diabetes into seven clear goals, each one designed to help you make important changes to your current eating habits without a lot of hassle.

What to Do

GOAL 1
Eat five+ servings of vegetables a day

The reason couldn't be simpler or clearer: People who eat more vegetables weigh less, have better blood sugar control, and slash their risk for diabetes-related diseases. These are all good reasons to make lunch a lavish salad, bite into baby carrots smeared with peanut butter for a snack, and invite two or even three vegetables over for dinner tonight.

GOAL 2
Cut your refined carbohydrates by half

Carbohydrates make blood sugar rise. Of course, they are also your body's main source of fuel. The solution: Choose your carbs carefully. Slash your intake of processed grains such as white rice and starchy vegetables such as potatoes, and focus on foods that give you a big nutrition bang for your carb buck without sending your sugar soaring.

GOAL 3
Eat three servings of fruit a day

Fruits have almost all the health advantages that vegetables bring, and they taste so good! Yes, fruit contains sugar. But it's chock-full of fiber and disease-fighting nutrients and doesn't contain a lot of calories, so it's perfect for helping you shed a few extra pounds. Nothing's off-limits; just keep an eye on your blood sugar and enjoy!

GOAL 4
Include lean protein at every meal

Protein has the unique ability to keep your stomach satisfied. Eating lean protein at every meal—fish, beans, eggs, lean meat and poultry, and low-fat dairy—helps keep blood sugar low, cuts between-meal cravings, and even helps preserve calorie-burning muscle while you're losing weight. We'll help you avoid protein pitfalls and fit this important nutrient into difficult meals such as breakfast.

What to Record

1. YOUR INTAKE OF KEY FOODS

During your 12-week challenge record how well you did against the seven eating goals on the habit trackers beginning on page 146. If you want a better understanding of your dietary strengths and weaknesses, keep a food diary during Week 1. You'll find a blank template on page 180.

2. THE NUMBER OF TIMES PER DAY YOU EAT IN RESPONSE TO STRESS, BOREDOM, OR HABIT

Emotional and mindless eating are major sources of excess calories, fat, and sugar, pack on pounds, and make blood sugar difficult to control. During your 12 week challenge you'll record every day how many times you ate not because you were hungry but in response to a mood or because food was in front of you. Gaining awareness of this type of eating is the key to overcoming it.

3. A MEAL PLAN FOR EVERY WEEK

Sit down once a week and fill out your weekly meal plan and shopping list using the templates on pages 176-177. This is a great time to pull out the calendar and look ahead for challenges: Will you have to eat on the run one night as you rush from work to an event? A good plan is all about adjusting for real life so that you stay on track.

Before You Begin

1 Take the quiz on page 28
It will help you assess your current eating habits and the state of your pantry, refrigerator, and freezer. Answer as honestly as you can—the info will help you find strengths as well as obstacles you may not have realized are standing in the way of better diabetes control.

2 Learn how to right-size portions.
If you're accustomed to heaping your plate full of pasta, take some time to study the Visual Guide to Portions on page 73 to understand how much you should really be eating

3 Stock up on healthy foods.
Does your pantry need an upgrade? Is your freezer packed with ice cream and popsicles, but a little short on frozen vegetables and boneless chicken breasts? Check out the kitchen makeover on page 174 and the grocery checklist on page 183 so you'll be ready to put a healthy meal on the table in a snap.

 GOAL 5

Trade good fat for bad

The key fat in hamburger meat, ice cream, and cheese is not only bad for your heart, it's bad for your diabetes. The same goes for trans fat, found in processed foods that contain hydrogenated oil. But that doesn't mean all fat is bad. On the Eat plan you'll enjoy plenty of it in the form of sugar-controlling "good" fats found in nuts, avocados, flaxseed, fish, and heart-healthy oils.

 GOAL 6

Use the Plate Approach for perfect portions

Could your dinner plate hold the key to right-sizing your portions? Yes! With our Plate Approach you won't have to measure or weigh foods at home to avoid portion distortion and overeating. This simple, proven method helps people with diabetes lose more weight and gain better blood sugar control. It's that easy and that effective.

GOAL 7

Plan your meals

If you know ahead of time what's for dinner, you'll be less tempted to turn to takeout or meals from a box. And planning and cooking meals at home gives you your best opportunity to follow the six other goals. You'll also know exactly what you need at the grocery store, so you're less likely to pick up snack foods, sweets, processed foods, and items high in saturated fat.

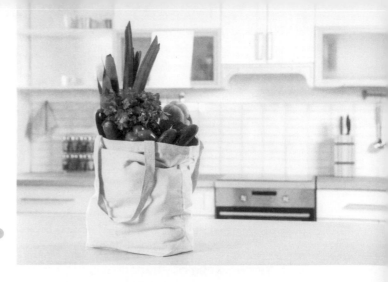

The Quiz

Do you pile your plate with vegetables or with fatty meat and mashed potatoes? Is your kitchen stocked with foods that spell success for people with diabetes or with tempting snacks and processed items that will thwart your best efforts to eat three healthy meals a day? This quiz will help uncover your strengths and weaknesses in two areas: your current eating habits and the foods you keep stocked in your kitchen.

Scan to find the quiz online.

Part One Your Diet

1. What's the star of most of your lunches and dinners?

a. Meat
b. Starch (pasta, potatoes, bread, rice, or corn)
c. Vegetables (except potatoes or corn)

2. Not counting potatoes and corn, how much room do vegetables usually occupy on your plate?

a. No room—I eat only potatoes and corn
b. About a quarter of the plate
c. Half of the plate or more

3. What is your usual choice when eating bread?

a. White bread
b. "Wheat" bread made mostly of white flour
c. 100% whole-grain bread

4. When it comes to vegetables, I:

a. Eat mashed potatoes, corn, or French fries, period
b. Force myself and my family to eat one green, red, or orange veggie at dinner
c. Love 'em and have no problem eating a rainbow of different colors

5. How often do you eat salads?

a. Salads are boring or too complicated to prepare, so I rarely eat them
b. Only when I go to a restaurant
c. Several times per week

6. Which of these fats do you usually use or cook with?

a. Butter or margarine containing hydrogenated oil
b. Margarine without hydrogenated oil, or corn oil
c. Olive, avocado, or canola oil

7. How often do you consume low-fat milk, cheese, or yogurt?

a. Rarely or never
b. Once a day
c. Two or three times a day

8. On average, how many soft drinks do you have each day?

a. Three or more
b. One or two
c. None

Your Score

Give yourself 1 point for every "a," 2 points for every "b," and 3 points for every "c." Add your points together.

20-24 points
Congratulations!
You're already following the type of eating plan that helps control blood sugar, keeps your weight in check, and lowers your odds for diabetes complications. The Eat plan will give you new ways to enjoy the foods you already love. We've also got smart strategies for dealing with your next challenge: sticking with the same strategies when you eat out.

16-20 points
A good start with room for improvement.
You probably need to invite more fruits, vegetables, and whole grains over to your dinner plate and choose higher-calorie foods and refined carbohydrates less often. Start this week and you'll be amazed how fast you see results in your blood sugar and on the scale. Finding smart, easy ways to add a variety of healthy foods—cooked in healthy ways—to your plate can transform this from a boring job into a pleasure. We'll show you how.

9-15 points
It's time for a change.
Your diet relies heavily on processed foods, refined carbohydrates, meats, and the empty calories in soft drinks—all of which get in the way of easy blood sugar control and maintaining a healthy body weight. Give yourself a big pat on the back for picking up this book, and get ready for delicious, healthy eating that will help you keep your blood sugar and weight under control.

8-10 points
Start the Eat plan today!
We suspect your diet is contributing to high blood sugar, stubborn extra pounds, and perhaps even early signs of diabetes complications such as high blood pressure, high cholesterol, and other problems. Pay special attention to the proven healthy-eating advice in this chapter, and talk with your doctor about arranging an appointment with a registered dietitian or certified diabetes educator to help you incorporate healthy eating strategies into your day.

Should You Supplement?

You're eating right, you're exercising—is there more you can do to protect your health? You bet! These three supplements can help protect your heart, guard against brittle bones and high blood pressure, and plug the occasional nutritional deficit. You'll notice that we're not suggesting any high-dose, single-vitamin or single-mineral supplements (with the exception of calcium). A growing stack of research suggests that approach is ineffective and can be downright dangerous for protecting health.

1. Multivitamin A multi can't make up for a poor diet, but it may help fill in nutritional gaps—especially for nutrients that become more difficult to absorb as we age. For people with diabetes, multivitamins can provide critical nutrients, such as magnesium, which many diabetics are deficient in, and chromium, which may help improve blood sugar and cholesterol levels, as well as B vitamins, which help protect the heart and nerves.

What to Take If you menstruate, look for a multivitamin that contains iron. If you don't, choose one without it. Make sure it contains 400 mcg of folic acid and 400 IU of vitamin D, as well as no more than 100 percent to 150 percent of the recommended daily value for other vitamins and minerals.

Note: Take with meals for best absorption.

2. Calcium Calcium protects the bones and helps keep blood pressure in check.

What to Take The recommended dosage is 600 mg twice a day. Calcium citrate is easier than other forms for people over 65 to digest.

3. Vitamin D Deficiency in this vitamin has been linked to an increased risk for diabetes, insulin resistance, and metabolic syndrome. Ask your doctor to have your D status checked.

What to Take The recommended daily dose is 15 mcg (600 IU), though your physician might prescribe more if your blood test reveals a severe deficiency.

Part Two | Your Kitchen

1. What are the first three things you see when you open your refrigerator door?

- ▲ Full-fat or 2% milk
- ● Nonfat or 1% milk and/or nonfat yogurt
- ▲ Full-fat cheese
- ● 100% fruit juice
- ● Fresh vegetables and fruits
- ● Meats such as extra-lean ground beef, ground skinless chicken or turkey, pork tenderloins
- ▲ Meats such as ground beef, T-bone steak, sausage, and chicken thighs
- ● Chicken breasts
- ▲ Soda (including diet soda), sweetened tea, or other sweetened drinks
- ▲ Regular mayonnaise and creamy salad dressings

2. What are the first three things you see when you open the freezer?

- ● Well-balanced frozen smart meals rich in protein, fiber, veggies, and whole grains
- ▲ Large-portioned, highly refined frozen meals such as mac 'n cheese and fried chicken
- ▲ Frozen pizza and/or French fries or deep-fried potatoes
- ▲ Frozen fish, breaded
- ● Frozen fish fillets, not breaded, no sauce
- ▲ Ice cream
- ● Frozen vegetables and/or fruits

3. Do you have fresh fruit in your house right now?

- ● Yes
- ▲ No

4. How many different packaged snack foods (chips, crackers, cookies, pretzels and etc.) do you have in your pantry right now?

- ● None
- ● One or two
- ▲ Three or more

5. Which of these are in your pantry right now?

- ● Canned beans
- ● Low-sodium canned soups and broths
- ▲ White rice, white pasta, white noodles
- ● Brown rice and other whole grains such as barley or bulgur
- ● Whole-grain pasta or noodles
- ▲ Fruit canned in heavy syrup
- ● Fruit canned in juice or extra-light syrup
- ▲ Peanut butter (or another nut butter) or unsalted nuts

Your Score

Add up the number of green circles you chose. The more circles, the closer your kitchen is to being ready for you to begin the plan.

11-16
Gold star kitchen!
Your cupboards, refrigerator, and freezer contain mostly diabetes-friendly foods such as whole grains, beans, fruit, vegetables, lean meat, fish, and low-fat or fat-free dairy products. We'll show you how to use even more of them in fast, delicious ways.

5-10
Your kitchen's sending mixed messages.
Too often, your kitchen sabotages your efforts to control your blood sugar and maintain a healthy weight. You have healthy foods here (give yourself a pat on the back!) but you may find yourself choosing unhealthy options because they're so tempting. Follow our kitchen makeover on page 174 for advice on what to keep and what to toss.

0-4
Your kitchen is hazardous to your health.
The foods in your house are contributing to your diabetes and dangerous belly fat around your middle. Turn to page 174 to make over your kitchen, and use the shopping list on page 183 to restock with foods that will help you follow the Eat plan with ease.

How to Keep a Food Diary

The better you understand the way you're really eating right now—and why—the better you'll be able to identify your strengths, downfalls, and biggest opportunities for improvement. During the 12-Week Challenge, you'll jot down a few details about your meals but if you want to go deeper, track what you're eating for the first week using the template on page 180. Write down:

• Everything you eat and drink and how much.

• The time you eat it, as well as the circumstances, such as "dinner at home," "popcorn at the movies," or "I was tired and cranky this morning so I gave in to the doughnuts at work."

At the end of the week, look over your diary for patterns. You may find that you consume more food than you realized in the form of late-night snacks, or beverages such as juice, soda, lattes, or beer. Also look critically to see how well your eating habits match up with the Eat goals, and figure out where they fall short. Are your breakfasts full of carbs but no protein? Are you getting anywhere near five servings of veggies a day? It's amazing what you'll learn when you look at your diet in black and white.

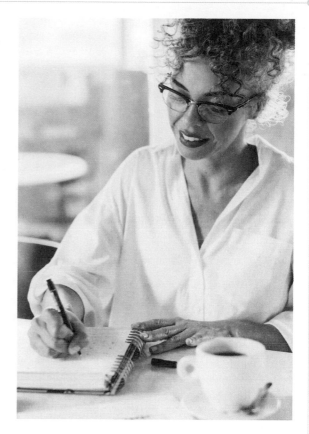

DATE May 23	TIME	WHAT I ATE/DRANK	NOTES
Breakfast	7 am	3 scrambled eggs; 2 slices toast; 1 Tbsp. butter; 6 oz. OJ	Feeling rushed
Lunch	1:30 pm	Sandwich: 3 oz. turkey, 3 oz. cheese, 2 slices bread, 1/2 tsp. mayo; apple; 8 oz. potato chips; 1 12-oz. cola	Ate at desk; really hungry
Dinner	7:30 pm	3 BBQ chicken thighs; 1 corn on cob; 1 cup watermelon chunks; 1 12-oz. beer	

GOAL 1

Eat five+ servings of vegetables a day

RIGHT OFF THE BAT, we know you're probably thinking, "Wow, that sounds like a lot of vegetables." So before we go any further, we want to clear up the confusion over what exactly a serving is. It's probably less than you think. See "What's in a Veggie Serving" on page 35. If you're really not used to eating vegetables at all, start with a modest goal of one more serving than you are currently eating. Once you're comfortable with that, add another serving, until you reach five a day. Once you get used to eating five servings a day, look for ways to bump that up to seven. There's new evidence that getting seven vegetable servings a day is even better for your health.

From juicy red peppers to springy green beans, from meaty portobello mushrooms to crunchy broccoli, vegetables are the ideal food for people with diabetes. Low in fat and calories, they're packed with fiber, vitamins, minerals, and other powerful nutrients that fight disease, pamper your blood sugar, and help you maintain a healthy weight. And let's face it—if you're eating more vegetables, you're eating less of everything else, including fatty meat, carbohydrate foods, and junk food. Now you know why this goal is number one on the Eat plan.

Over and over again, researchers have found that eating more vegetables is a key strategy for losing weight and keeping it off. Vegetables make you feel full and satisfied for very few calories. The simple truth: The more vegetables you eat, the less you'll weigh. In one study at Pennsylvania State University, women who started a meal with a low-calorie salad and then ate a pasta dish ate about 12 percent fewer calories in total than women who skipped the salad and started right in on the pasta. In another study, adding about six ounces of vegetables (in this case, carrots and spinach) to dinner helped people feel fuller on fewer calories.

STEP ONE

Shop with Intent

No veggies in the fridge, freezer or pantry? Then you'll be forced to eat a dinner that's virtually veggie-free or go for chips, cookies, candy, cheese, or whatever else is on hand when you're hungry and need a snack. The first rule of eating more vegetables, then, is to make sure they're ready and waiting, in the most user-friendly forms possible.

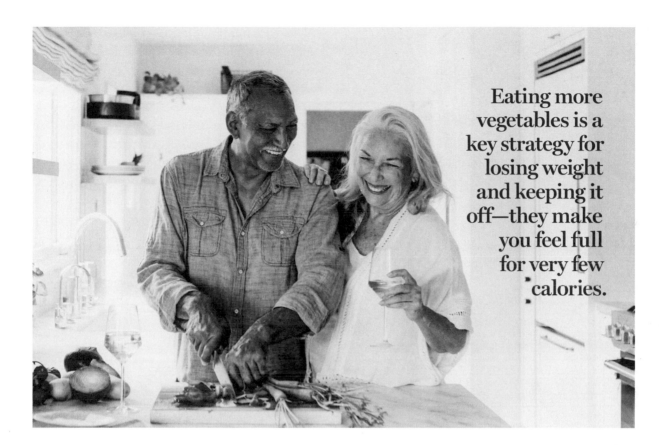

Eating more vegetables is a key strategy for losing weight and keeping it off—they make you feel full for very few calories.

Take advantage of prepared produce. We usually don't recommend prepared foods. They're more expensive and often high in artificial flavorings, sugars, and sodium. But when it comes to prepared veggies—bagged salads, prewashed spinach, peeled and diced butternut squash, washed and chopped kale, riced cauliflower—we're all for it. Numerous studies find that we're more likely to use bagged salads and other produce than produce that requires more preparation.

Buy "now" and "later" fresh vegetables. When you grocery shop, choose just a few vegetables from the produce section that you can use up over the next four or five days, such as lettuce, spinach, and tomatoes. Invest the rest of your fresh-veggie budget in types that keep well, such as carrots, celery, cab-

bage, onions, winter squash, sweet potatoes, and garlic. That way, vegetables won't languish in your fridge, and you'll always have produce on hand even when it's tough to get to the store for more perishable items.

Stock your pantry and freezer with canned and frozen vegetables. They can be as nutritious as fresh veggies because they're picked and frozen at their peak, when they are the most nutrient-rich. Frozen vegetables are flash-frozen, which seals in the nutrients until the veggies are thawed. Don't worry about losing nutrients that leach into water in cans: The amounts are small, and you lose nothing if you use the water in dishes such as soup. Just be sure to choose naked veggies—those without sauce or cheese.

STEP TWO
Aim for Variety

We have a tendency to lump all vegetables together as if they were a single food. But vegetables can be sweet, bitter, or bland; big or small; and green, orange, yellow, red, brown, and every shade and flavor in between. Given the sheer bounty of natural foods at your disposal, how do you decide which to eat?

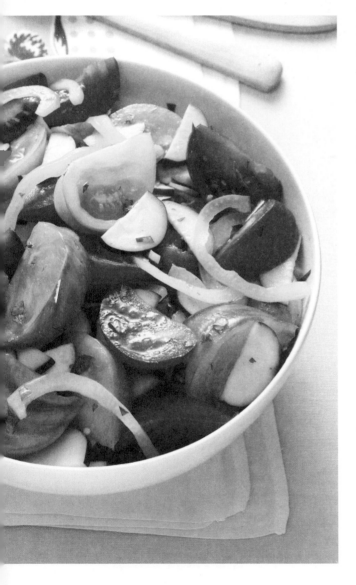

The first thing to do is to vote with your taste buds and eat produce you like. If you tend to eat only one veggie, such as frozen green beans, try to vary your routine. This will help ensure that you get all the nutrients you need. A serving of broccoli may have dozens of powerhouse nutrients—but not necessarily the same ones as a serving of asparagus.

Getting the variety of nutrients found in a variety of vegetables is important for controlling blood sugar and cutting your risk for diabetes complications such as heart disease and high blood pressure. In one British study, people with the highest blood levels of vitamin C were less likely to have high A1C scores, a long-term indicator of high blood sugar. In another study, people with the highest blood levels of beta-carotene—found in carrots and winter squash—had 32 percent lower insulin levels (suggesting better blood sugar control) than those with the lowest levels. Dark, leafy greens such as spinach, Swiss chard, bok choy, collards, and mustard greens provide zinc, a mineral that protects insulin-producing beta cells in the pancreas. Zinc is lost in the urine when blood sugar is too high, so replacing it is vitally important if you have diabetes.

Ready to munch and crunch?

Start by choosing veggies with star nutritional power. Vivid color is one indicator of nutrient richness in vegetables. Often, these nutrients are especially helpful for people with diabetes. Try these versatile superstars:

Broccoli. Big on volume and small on calories, broccoli is a great way to bulk up carbohydrate-rich dishes (think pasta, casseroles, and baked potatoes) to blunt their effect on your blood sugar and your waistline. This classic is one of the best food sources of chromium, a mineral required for insulin to function normally (remember, insulin helps the body use up blood sugar so there's less in the bloodstream). One cup of broccoli provides almost half of your daily chromium requirement. Fiber, at a hearty four grams per stalk, is also part of broccoli's "benefits package."

Carrots. Don't believe the hype that carrots raise your blood sugar rapidly. Chalk up that myth to a problem with the Glycemic Index, a system that preceded the more accurate Glycemic Load. While the type of sugar carrots contain is transformed into blood sugar very rapidly, the amount of sugar in carrots is extremely low. Thank goodness, because they're one of the richest sources of beta-carotene, which is linked to a lower risk of diabetes. Like most vegetables, carrots are also a good source of beneficial fiber. By the way, carrots won't help you throw away your reading glasses, but they will help protect against two sight-robbing conditions: macular degeneration and cataracts.

Spinach, kale, and other dark, leafy greens. Thanks to rich stores of carotenoids (including beta-carotene and other "carotenes"), these yummy greens are among the most antioxidant-rich vegetables on earth. Antioxidants are powerful weapons against diabetes-related complications, including heart disease and nerve damage, not to mention cancer. They're also loaded with potassium and magnesium, which help keep blood pressure in check.

Sweet potatoes. These potatoes are packed with nutrients and disease-fighting fiber, almost 40 percent of which is soluble fiber, the kind that helps lower blood sugar and cholesterol. Sweet potatoes are extraordinarily rich in carotenoids, orange and yellow pigments that play a role in helping the body respond to insulin. They're also full of the natural plant compound chlorogenic acid, which may help reduce insulin resistance.

What's in a Veggie Serving?

Here's the definition of a serving from the National Cancer Institute. All varieties of fruits and vegetables—fresh, frozen, canned, dried, and 100 percent juice—count. Measure out some of these in your kitchen so you can see how reasonable a serving size is.

- ½ cup raw, cooked, canned, or frozen vegetables
- ¾ cup (6 ounces) 100 percent vegetable juice
- ½ cup cooked or canned legumes (beans and peas)
- 1 cup raw, leafy vegetables such as lettuce and spinach

STEP THREE

Have at Least One Vegetable Side Dish at Dinner

Make it an automatic rule: You will have at least one vegetable on your plate at dinner—and lunch whenever you can. This can be as easy as tossing baby carrots or cherry tomatoes into a zip-close bag. These strategies can help make the most of the great flavors and textures in these amazing foods.

Give veggies a roast. Here is one of the great side dishes—easy to make, delicious to eat, and amazingly healthy. Plus, it tastes surprisingly sweet and lasts well, meaning you can make large batches and serve throughout the week. Cut root vegetables such as parsnips, turnips, rutabagas, carrots, and onions into inch-thick chunks and arrange in a single layer on a sheet pan. Drizzle with olive oil and sprinkle with salt, freshly ground pepper, and fresh or dried herbs. Roast in a 450°F oven until soft, about 45 minutes, turning once.

Throw 'em on the grill. Peppers, zucchini, asparagus, onions, eggplant—even tomatoes—all taste amazingly good when grilled. Generally, all you need to do is coat them with olive oil and throw them on. Turn every few minutes and remove when they start to soften. Or thread chunks of veggies on to a bamboo or metal skewer and turn frequently. You can also buy grilling baskets that keep the veggies from falling through the slats in the grill.

Buy a vegetable steamer. It's one of the healthiest ways to cook vegetables because nutrients aren't lost in the water. Choose a metal or bamboo steamer basket, fill it with veggies, place over a saucepan of rapidly simmering water, cover, and cook for 5 to 10 minutes. It's that simple.

STEP FOUR

Sneak in Veggies at Every Opportunity

The average American is lucky to get two servings of vegetables a day—far less than the five we're suggesting. This gap pretty much captures America's health problems in a nutshell. If we ate more vegetables and fewer processed foods, we'd lose weight, clean our arteries, balance our blood sugar, and shut down a large number of hospitals. But getting from two servings a day to five doesn't come without planning or effort. We're here to help. Here's how to sneak more veggies into your daily diet.

Breakfast, Lunch, and Snacks

Sneak vegetables into breakfast. One reason we don't get enough vegetables is that many of us consider them merely a side dish to dinner. But

Vegetable Seasoning Guide

Think beyond butter when it comes to seasoning vegetables. Try these delicious combinations:

VEGETABLE	BEST HERBS, SPICES, AND FLAVORINGS
ASPARAGUS	Lemon, garlic, oregano
BROCCOLI	Garlic, soy sauce, mustard, dark sesame oil
CARROTS	Lemon, orange, curry powder, ginger, dill, raspberry vinegar
CAULIFLOWER	Basil, curry powder
EGGPLANT	Basil, garlic, crushed tomato
GREEN BEANS	Garlic, soy sauce, sesame seeds
MUSHROOMS	Parsley, thyme, green onions, chives, sherry, balsamic vinegar
PEAS	Mint, garlic
SPINACH	Garlic, soy sauce, sea salt, nutmeg, balsamic vinegar
SUMMER SQUASH	Lemon, rosemary, tomato, garlic, basil
TOMATO	Basil, garlic, oregano, balsamic vinegar, Parmesan cheese

eggs are perfect vegetable vehicles. Make egg scrambles a regular breakfast, using a scrambled egg to hold together lightly sautéed vegetables such as peppers, mushrooms, zucchini, asparagus, or onions.

Build a sandwich that has more lettuce and tomato than meat. Stack the meat filler in the sandwich to no higher than the thickness of a standard slice of bread. Then pile on low-calorie lettuce and slices of tomatoes to the combined height of both slices of bread. Presto: Your sandwich tower has the height of the Empire State Building yet the svelteness of the Eiffel Tower.

Experiment with zucchini. Chop and drain, then mix into ground turkey or beef burger patties. Sneak it into baked muffins and breads. Spiralize it and use it in place of pasta.

Open a can of low-sodium soup and add veggies. Toss in a bag of precut broccoli and carrots, either fresh or frozen, and voilà! You have a superfast and easy lunch or dinner entrée, ready to be flavored with your preferred spices, herbs, or hot sauce. As the soup simmers, it will simultaneously cook the veggies, boosting the dish's nutritional value and fiber.

Eat vegetables as if they were fruit. Half a cucumber, a whole tomato, a stalk of celery, or a long, fresh carrot are as pleasant to munch on as an apple. It may not seem typical, but who cares? A whole vegetable makes a terrific snack.

Dinner and Dessert

Start each dinner with a mixed green salad before you serve the main course. Not only will it help you eat more veggies, but by filling your stomach first with a nutrient-rich, low-calorie salad, you'll have just a bit less room for the higher-calorie items that follow. For an instant, perfectly dressed salad, open a bag of prewashed,

Five Things
to Do with Broccoli

- Chop spears and add them to stir-fries.

- Steam just long enough for the broccoli to turn brilliant green. Eat the softer-but-crunchy spears as finger food for a taste that's different from that of either raw or fully cooked broccoli.

- Add raw or lightly steamed to a garden salad or a vegetable-and-dip tray.

- Sauté with a little garlic and oil and top with a dusting of Parmesan for a quick, low-calorie side dish.

- Steam, and make soup by adding to chicken broth along with a bit of garlic and some onions, then pureeing. For a creamier version, add fat-free evaporated milk.

precut romaine lettuce or mixed greens, add a tablespoon of olive oil and a splash of lemon juice or balsamic vinegar, and shake.

Put a plate of raw vegetables in the center of the table. Nearly everyone likes carrot sticks, celery sticks, cucumber slices, string beans, cherry tomatoes, and red, green, and yellow pepper strips. They're healthy, they have virtually no calories, a satisfying crunch, and can substantially cut your consumption of the more calorie-dense main course.

Once a week, have an entrée salad. A salade niçoise is a good example: mixed greens, steamed green beans, boiled potatoes, sliced hard-boiled egg, and tuna drizzled with vinaigrette. Serve with crusty whole-grain bread. Bon appétit!

Fill your spaghetti sauce with vegetables. Then replace half the pasta you normally eat with more vegetables. Open a jar of low-sodium prepared sauce and add in string beans, peas, corn,

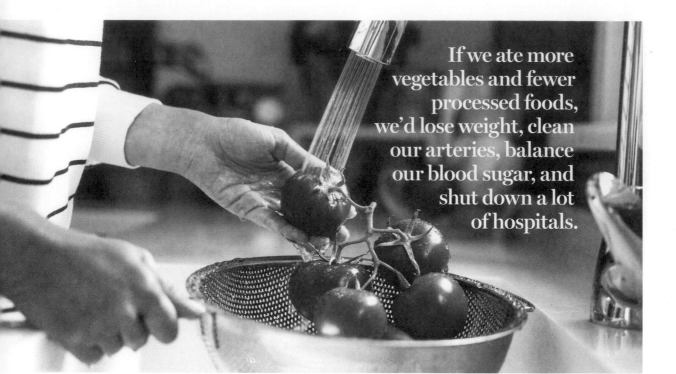

If we ate more vegetables and fewer processed foods, we'd lose weight, clean our arteries, balance our blood sugar, and shut down a lot of hospitals.

bell peppers, mushrooms, tomatoes and more. Like it chunky? Cut them in big pieces. Don't want to know they're there? Shred or puree them with a bit of sauce in the blender, then add. And don't stop there. Steamed broccoli or green beans, or baked spaghetti squash (use a fork to remove the spaghetti-like strands), are filling and delicious replacements for the mounds of pasta that often find their way onto our plates.

Order your pizza with extra veggies. Instead of the same old pepperoni, do your blood sugar and digestion a favor and ask for half the cheese and double the sauce, and add toppings such as artichoke hearts, broccoli, hot peppers, and other vegetables many pizza joints stock.

Puree cooked veggies into soup. Potatoes, carrots, winter squash, cauliflower, and broccoli—just about any cooked (or leftover) vegetable can be made into a creamy, comforting soup. Here's a simple recipe: In a medium saucepan, sauté 1 cup finely chopped onion in one tablespoon vegetable oil until tender. Combine the onion in a blender or food processor with 2 or more cups of cooked vegetables and puree until smooth. Return puree to saucepan and thin with broth or low-fat milk. Simmer and season to taste.

Go meatless one day a week. You can do this by merely substituting the meat serving with a vegetable serving (suggestion: make it a crunchy, strong-flavored vegetable such as broccoli or a hearty one such as squash or mushrooms). To ensure that you get enough protein, consider peas, lentils, and other beans and legumes. Soy foods, nuts, and eggs are all also great sources of protein. Get a good plant-based cookbook or check out one of the many plant-forward cooking sites online to find vegetarian and vegan main dish recipes to add to your repertoire. You can start with the Fiery Stuffed Poblanos on page 219 or the Easy Vegetable Lasagna on page 224. If you're already eating meatless once a week, add another vegetarian day to your week.

Use salsa liberally. Salsa shouldn't be just for chips. It's too tasty and healthy not to be used on everything: baked potatoes, rice, chicken breasts, fish, sandwiches, eggs, steak, even bread. Be careful with store-bought salsa, though; some brands can have significant amounts of added sugar and salt. Luckily, it's easy to make your own—just chop some fresh tomatoes, onions, and garlic, season with salt and pepper, and add a little lime juice. Experiment with different combinations of fruits, vegetables and seasonings. Chopped yellow squash, zucchini or bell peppers add body; chopped pineapple, mango or peach add a little sweetness; chopped jalapeno peppers or chili powder add a nice kick if you like a little heat.

Throw a bag of preshredded carrots and cabbage into your next soup, salad, or casserole. Available in the produce department, these coleslaw ingredients add flavor, color, and lots of vitamins and minerals.

Use vegetables as sauces. How about pureed roasted red peppers seasoned with herbs and a bit of lemon juice, then drizzled over fish? Or puree butternut or acorn squash with carrots, grated ginger, and dollop of unsweetened applesauce for a yummy topping for chicken or turkey. Cooked vegetables are easily converted into sauces. It just takes a little ingenuity and a blender.

Bake some pumpkin pudding for dessert. It's easy—and delicious! In a bowl, beat together ½ cup egg white (or egg substitute), 1 can pumpkin, 2 packets zero-calorie sweetener, 1 teaspoon cinnamon,

Eat Your ABCs

Knowing tasty ways to cook a vegetable makes you all the more likely to eat it. Try these tips.

Asparagus Roast them in the oven with a little olive oil. Delicious! Or make instant asparagus soup by pureeing cooked asparagus, heating it with a little milk, and adding chopped parsley or tarragon.

Broccoli Overcooking can degrade some of broccoli's nutrients, so steam florets lightly, shorten cooking time in the microwave, or quickly stir-fry them in a small amount of olive oil. To eat them almost raw but cooked enough to soften them up, blanch broccoli spears in boiling water for about 3 minutes.

Brussels sprouts The stems are tougher than the leaves, so cut an "X" across the base of each sprout before steaming to allow heat inside the core to soften it. For the mildest taste, choose frozen baby Brussels sprouts. For the best flavor, cook them lightly so they're still a little crisp.

Cauliflower Instead of mashed potatoes, try this tasty cauliflower puree. Boil a head of cauliflower cut into florets, one diced peeled potato, and six peeled garlic cloves until tender. Drain and puree (in batches) in a food processor and thin with enough warm milk to make it velvety. Drizzle olive oil on top and season with salt and pepper. (Or try the recipe for Cauliflower Mash on page 229.) Alternatively try making riced cauliflower. Simply cut up the cauliflower into chunks and pulse in the food processor until it resembles grains of rice. Then saute lightly to use in place of rice.

½ teaspoon nutmeg, and ½ cup fat-free evaporated milk. Pour into four eight-ounce custard cups coated with cooking spray. Place on a cookie sheet. Bake uncovered at 400°F for 8 to 10 minutes. Reduce heat to 300°F and bake for another 30 minutes until a knife inserted comes out clean. Serve warm or cold.

Top 20 Foods for Diabetes

Just about any good-for-you food fits into the Eat plan, including every fresh fruit and green (and red, orange, and yellow) vegetable under the sun. But these 20 foods have properties that make them extra-appealing for people with diabetes.

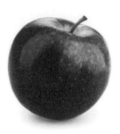

1 Apples This year-round favorite is loaded with soluble fiber—number one for blunting blood sugar swings. A medium apple dishes up an impressive 4 grams of fiber, mostly pectin, known for its ability to lower cholesterol. Go for whole, unpeeled fruit but wash it well.

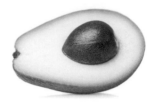

2 Avocado Rich, creamy, and packed with good fat, avocado slows digestion to help keep blood sugar from spiking after a meal. A diet high in the fat it contains may even help reverse insulin resistance, which translates to steadier blood sugar over the long term.

3 Barley Barley may just be the perfect substitute for rice. Soluble fiber and other compounds in barley slow the digestion and absorption of blood sugar dramatically. Choosing this grain instead of a refined grain such as white rice can reduce the rise in blood sugar after a meal by almost 70 percent—and can keep your blood sugar lower and steadier for hours.

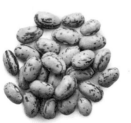

4 Beans The soluble fiber in all types of beans puts a lid on high blood sugar. And because they're rich in protein, beans can stand in for meat in salads and even main dishes. Best of all, you only have to open a can.

5 Fish Serve up salmon, mackerel, or other fish and you'll be managing your diabetes by fighting inflammation in your body, and by getting good fats, which help steady blood sugar. You'll also slash your risk of heart disease, the most deadly diabetes complication.

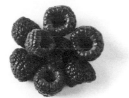

6 Berries Full of fiber and especially rich in all-important antioxidants, berries are a low-calorie, low-sugar way to satisfy a sweet tooth.

7 Broccoli Filling, fibrous, and full of antioxidants (including a day's worth of vitamin C in one serving), broccoli is also rich in chromium, which plays an important role in long-term blood sugar control.

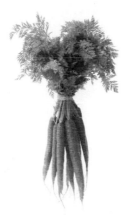

8 Carrots They're one of nature's richest sources of beta-carotene, which is linked to a lower risk of diabetes. And raw carrots (dipped in a little peanut butter or hummus) make perfect snacks.

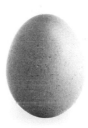

10 Eggs Eggs are an excellent, inexpensive source of high-quality protein. An egg or two won't raise your blood sugar (or cholesterol in most people) and can keep you feeling full and satisfied for hours after a meal.

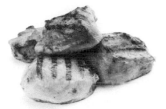

9 Chicken and turkey White meat chicken is one of the leanest, lowest-calorie protein sources money can buy. Turkey breast is even lower in calories. Ground skinless turkey breast is a smart substitute for ground beef.

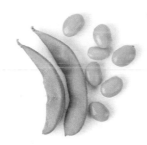

11 Soy foods Compounds called isoflavones in soy foods such as tofu, tempeh and edamame help to lower cholesterol and decrease blood sugar levels. They can also be a great source of fiber and plant-based protein. Just be sure to stick with minimally processed soy foods.

continued >>>

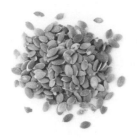

12 Seeds Seeds of all types—pumpkin, sunflower, sesame, chia, and beyond—are filled with good fats, protein, and fiber that work together to keep blood sugar low and to stave off heart disease. Flaxseed is a good source of magnesium, a mineral that's key to good blood sugar control because it helps cells use insulin.

13 Milk and yogurt These are rich in protein and calcium, which studies show may help people lose weight. And diets that include plenty of dairy may fight insulin resistance, a core problem behind diabetes. Go low-fat or fat-free when you eat or drink dairy.

14 Nuts Where else can you get a protein-rich, fiber-heavy snack that's also loaded with good fat? Nuts couldn't be any friendlier to your blood sugar. Just stick with a small handful or, for nut butter, two thumb-sized portions.

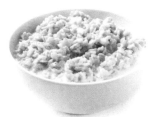

15 Oatmeal Thanks to its soluble fiber, it's even better for your blood sugar than starting the day with a whole-grain cold cereal. And it's extraordinarily kind to your heart.

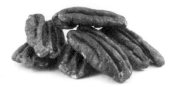

16 Olive oil Unlike butter, the good fat in olive oil won't increase insulin resistance and may even help reverse it, helping your body steady its own blood sugar. A touch of olive oil also slows the emptying of the stomach, so your meal is less likely to spike your blood sugar. And of course the oil is heart-friendly.

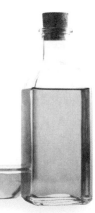

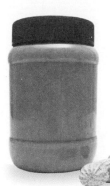

17 Peanut butter

A study at Purdue University found that eating peanut butter can dampen appetite for up to two hours longer than a low-fiber, high-carb snack, making this childhood favorite a grown-up weight-loss ally. Monounsaturated fats in peanut butter also help control blood sugar.

18 Sweet potatoes

Choose a baked sweet potato instead of a baked white potato, and your blood sugar will rise about 30 percent less. Sweet potatoes are packed with nutrients and disease-fighting fiber—almost 40 percent of which is soluble fiber, the kind that helps lower blood sugar and cholesterol.

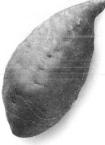

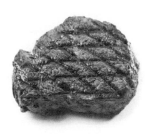

19 Beef

Yes, beef is a diabetes-friendly food, as long as you choose the leanest cuts and keep portions to a quarter of your plate. Getting enough protein in your meals helps keep you full and satisfied, and it helps you maintain muscle mass when you're losing weight, so that your metabolism keeps burning on high.

20 Whole-wheat bread

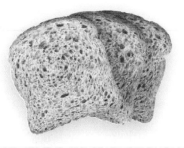

White bread is one of the five foods in our diets that raise blood sugar the most. Switch to whole wheat and you may improve your sensitivity to insulin, the hormone that manages blood sugar. In one study of 978 people, the higher their intake of whole grains, the greater their insulin sensitivity, which translates into better blood sugar control.

GOAL 2

Cut your refined carbohydrates by half

SIMPLY PUT, MOST AMERICANS eat way too many of the carbohydrates that send blood sugar soaring. We munch lots of potatoes, mostly fried. We consume enormous quantities of bread, most of it made with refined white flour that has little or no fiber. We eat a lot of rice, most of it white. We breakfast on pastries and muffins and snack on bags of potato chips and pretzels. And we wash it all down with sugar-sweetened sodas and fruit drinks. In fact, of all the extra daily calories we've taken to consuming over the past decade or two, nearly all come from one source: refined carbohydrates.

It's time to dial down the carbohydrate mania, the smart way.

Let's be clear: We're not talking about a "just say no" approach to carbohydrates. Your body needs the energy and nutrients found in grains, vegetables, dried beans, fruits, and milk (yes, all of these foods count—at least in part—as carbohydrates because they contain starches and/or sugars). Instead, we ask you to make a conscious effort to choose more whole grains and fewer refined grain products; eat smaller portions of grain-based carbs; and spend much more of your "carb budget" on vegetables and fresh fruit.

STEP ONE
Say "Less" to Refined Carbs

Reducing or eliminating just a few foods that spike blood sugar can make a huge difference when it comes to managing your diabetes. In many cases, you don't have to stop eating the food completely. Instead, you reduce your portion size and/or the number of times a day you seek out that food.

Skip the dinner rolls. Bread isn't bad for you, especially if it's whole grain. But if you had a sandwich at lunch or toast with your eggs at breakfast, that's probably all the bread you need for the day.

Buy smaller tortillas. Though a super-sized 13-inch tortilla checks in at 330 calories, an eight-inch one provides half that amount—but is still plenty for your taco or burrito.

Eat less rice, and choose carefully. Stick with one serving, or ½ cup, per meal. Your best choice when it comes to your blood sugar? Whole grain brown, red, or black rice. Bonus: mix in some riced cauliflower, which will help you make headway for Eat Goal #1.

Cut your pasta in half. Even white pasta has a lower glycemic load than bread because of the way the starch molecules are interwoven with protein molecules, making the starch in pasta harder to break down. That means pasta is relatively friendly to your blood sugar, especially if it's al dente. Still, it's best to avoid making pasta the dominant food on your plate. Have no more than a cup of pasta and bulk it up with sautéed peppers, mushrooms, spinach, or other vegetables.

Indulge in parsnip and carrot "fries." Cut down the length of parsnips and carrots to make long, thin strips. Place on a baking sheet, drizzle with olive oil, sprinkle with salt and pepper, and roast in a 400°F oven for about 40 minutes.

Say so long to soda. These beverages have zero nutritional value, but each 12-ounce serving of regular soda contains about 150 calories—virtually all of it sugar. (That's equivalent to nine packets of sugar!) And studies show that soda calories don't fill you up the way food does, so you end up consuming more calories throughout the day than you would if you got those 150 calories from something you could sink your teeth into. What else is there to drink? Plenty.

Water. It has zero calories and quenches thirst better than sugary drinks. Drink it liberally, since dehydration can raise blood sugar. Add a squeeze of lemon or lime juice to make it more interesting.

Sparkling water. Choose plain water or sugar-free, fruit-flavored varieties.

Iced tea. Make your own by steeping two tea bags in a tall glass of cold water. If you drink bottled iced tea, be sure it's sugar- and calorie-free.

Lemonade. Making your own with fresh lemon juice and sweetening it with a sugar substi-

Smart Substitutions

Each substitution raises blood sugar just half as much as the food it replaces.

FOOD	SUBSTITUTION
Cooked potatoes	Whole-grain pasta
Sugary breakfast cereal	High-fiber breakfast cereal
White bread	Coarse 100% whole-grain bread
Muffin	Apple
White rice	Pearled barley

tute cuts out the calories, saving more than 100 calories than with store-bought lemonade.

STEP TWO
Have Three to Six Servings of Whole Grains Every Day

The total number of grain-based carb servings you should aim for every day will depend on your own personal blood sugar patterns and the dietary advice you get from your doctor, registered dietitian, or certified diabetes educator. But almost certainly you should be eating more whole grains than you do now. A serving is small—one slice of 100 percent whole-grain bread or half a cup of cooked pasta or grains. Even so, most of us eat less than one serving a day.

Why should you go whole? It's simple. Eating more whole grains has been shown to cut heart disease risk by 25 percent in women and 18 percent in men (again, heart disease is the number one killer of people with diabetes). It also helps keep blood sugar steady. In one study of 978 people, the more whole grains people ate, the greater their insulin sensitivity, which translates into better blood sugar control.

And consider the weight-loss benefits: The famous Nurses' Health Study from the Harvard School of Public Health looked at more than 74,000 women and found that those who ate the most whole grains were a whopping 49 percent less likely to gain weight over a 12-year period than those who ate the least.

Whole grains contain all the parts of the grain—not just the starchy low-fiber center, but also the nutrient-rich germ layer and the fiber-rich bran

The Not-So-Sweet Truth About "Diabetic" Foods

Can you eat "sugar-free," "low-carb," and "diabetic" candies, cookies, and desserts to your heart's content? The surprising answer is no. You'd think sugar-free foods such as candy and soft drinks would have less impact on blood-glucose levels and waistlines than regular candy or soft drinks. But it's not that simple.

The sweeteners they contain—called sugar alcohols—have half the calories of sugar. Under food-labeling laws, products containing sugar alcohols are permitted to call themselves sugar-free. But in fact sweeteners such as maltitol, mannitol, sorbitol, and xylitol may not be sucrose (the technical name for regular sugar), but they do contain carbohydrates, each gram of which can raise blood glucose just as much as sugar does. They can also cause intestinal distress—from bloating and gassy rumbling to diarrhea. The products they're in often have just as many calories as regular goodies. Our advice: Pay no attention to "sugar-free" claims on the packaging. Look instead at a product's total carbohydrate count and calories. Then enjoy some fresh fruit!

layer on the outside. The result: You get antioxidants, vitamins, minerals, and a wide range of plant compounds that protect against chronic disease in many ways.

Many Americans just aren't used to eating whole grains and may not know where to begin. Fortunately, it's easy to do.

Start your day with a high-fiber cereal. A quick and simple way to get one of your daily servings of whole grains than starting your day with a whole-grain cereal. Look for a brand with the word "whole" in the first ingredient and at least 3 grams of fiber per serving. It's also important to look for cereals with low sugar content. That way, you'll control calories and stay off the blood sugar roller coaster that leads to midmorning hunger pangs and food cravings. (A British study recently found that eating sugary cereal actually led to overeating at lunch.) Top your cereal with berries to squeeze in a fruit serving. For protein, consider making a cereal parfait with plain Greek yogurt or Skyr, both of which are richer in protein than regular yogurt.

Buy bread and rolls with the word "whole" in the first ingredient. This is the simplest way to shift the balance from refined to whole-grain carbs in your diet. Don't be fooled by the marketing terms on the front of the label. For example, coloring a loaf of bread brown and calling it wheat bread doesn't make it whole wheat. Or saying a product is "made with wheat flour" could be true of both whole-wheat bread and angel food cake. If a product is truly whole grain, the label will list whole wheat, whole oats, or some other whole grain as the first ingredient on the label.

Switch pastas. Whole-wheat pasta is widely available, and it tastes better than ever. Also look for whole-wheat couscous, a type of pasta that

Since whole-grain pastas are higher in fiber, they have less impact on your blood sugar.

cooks in five minutes. For pasta that's even friendlier to your blood sugar, go with one of the many new high-fiber, high-protein options that have popped up on supermarket shelves. Some are multigrain pastas, made from grains such as oats, spelt, and barley in addition to durum wheat. Since these are higher in soluble fiber, they have less impact on your blood sugar than regular pasta. Some contain flaxseed as a source of heart-healthy omega-3 fatty acids. Some have added protein—40 or 50 percent more than regular pasta—from sources such as soy flour, milk solids, or egg whites. Some are made from lentils, chickpeas or other legumes. This also makes them more blood sugar friendly.

Use fibrous fixings. Bran cereal, oat bran, and wheat germ make good condiments when sprinkled over oatmeal, applesauce, cottage cheese, or yogurt. In recipes that call for bread crumbs, try oatmeal or whole-grain bread—toasted, then reduced to crumbs in your food processor.

Bake with the whole stuff. Give a boost to homemade baked goods by replacing one-third of the white flour with whole-wheat flour.

Set a brown rice rule. With six times more fiber than white rice, brown rice is packed with vitamins and minerals such as bone-building magnesium, immune-boosting selenium, and manganese, which helps keep up the body's natural defenses. Many restaurants also offer it, if you ask. Just be sure to keep your portion size to half a cup. While it's much better for you than white rice, even brown rice raises blood sugar quite a bit.

Try a variety of whole grains. Beyond oats, whole wheat and brown rice, many whole grains are on supermarket shelves these days. Experiment with barley, quinoa, farro, freekeh, millet, kamut, and teff, to name a few. Keep in mind that most whole grains either require soaking overnight or can take about 45 minutes to prepare, so start early or make a big batch and freeze meal-size portions.

One exception is bulgur, also known as kasha. Wheat grain that's been partially cooked by boiling or steaming, then dried and cracked, bulgur cooks in about 15 minutes—great for a weeknight dinner. You'll find bulgur in different textures. Coarse bulgur is used for pilaf and rice dishes, medium is used as breakfast cereal, and fine is used for tabbouleh (a Middle Eastern salad made with bulgur, chopped parsley, cucumbers, tomatoes, olive oil, and lemon juice). The finer the grain, the quicker bulgur cooks up.

Serve bulgur pilaf as a side dish. There are a million different recipes, some including dried

47

fruit and some with vegetables and/or herbs. Grab a good cookbook and take your pick. You can also enjoy bulgur in cold salads.

Stuff zucchini with extra-lean beef or pork mixed with bulgur.

Throw together some tabbouleh as an excellent, portable summertime lunch salad or side dish. Toss in chopped vegetables from your garden, such as tomatoes and cucumbers, and add some goat or feta cheese or chicken for extra protein.

Cook up hot bulgur cereal in salted water as you would oatmeal. Top with fresh fruit or with chopped walnuts, dried cranberries, cinnamon, and a drizzle of honey. Some manufacturers make bulgur cereals with extra ingredients, such as soy, which adds extra protein.

STEP THREE
Eat at Least One Food Rich in Soluble Fiber a Day

There are two types of fiber: soluble and insoluble. Most whole grains are rich in insoluble fiber, which passes through you undigested. Soluble fiber is the kind that dissolves in water. It's found in oats, barley, beans, fruits, and vegetables. Both are very good for you, but only soluble fiber will help you lower your blood sugar in a big way.

Researchers tested the two top grain sources of soluble fiber—oatmeal and barley—on overweight middle-aged women. On days when they ate oatmeal for breakfast, their blood sugar levels over the next three hours were about 30 percent lower than when they ate a sugar-laden pudding. On days they ate barley cereal, it was about 60 percent lower.

How does soluble fiber help control blood sugar? When it mixes with water it forms a gum.

Think of oatmeal. You can pick out the grains or flakes when it's dry, but once you cook it, it's one big mush. This gum forms a barrier between the digestive enzymes in your stomach and the starch molecules in the food—not just the oatmeal, but even in the toast you ate it with. So it takes longer for your body to convert the whole meal into blood sugar, and a slower rise in blood sugar is a good thing for your health.

Eating more foods rich in soluble fiber is a key strategy for lowering your blood sugar after meals. It will also improve your health in other ways. Oatmeal is famous for lowering cholesterol; it may also lower high levels of triglycerides as well as high blood pressure. There's even a health claim allowed on oatmeal: "Eating three grams of soluble fiber from oatmeal in a diet low in saturated fat and cholesterol may reduce the risk of heart disease."

To get more soluble fiber into your diet, start with these easy strategies.

Have oatmeal for breakfast. Stick with about a cup, and fill up the rest of your bowl with fresh fruit and a sprinkling of nuts. A steaming bowl of oatmeal—sprinkled with sugar-lowering cinnamon—is more than comfort food. Studies show that oats can reduce post-meal blood sugar and insulin levels in people with diabetes. Oats are also an excellent source of the mineral manganese, which plays a role in blood sugar metabolism.

Add oats while cooking. Make a batch of oat bran muffins and keep them on hand for tasty breakfast treats. And next time you make pancakes or waffles, replace up to one-third of the flour in the batter with oatmeal ground to a fine powder in the blender. Just don't substitute instant oats in a recipe that calls for quick-cooking or old-fashioned oats. The texture is different, and instant oats usually have other flavors added.

That's Easy!

Simply eating the right breakfast cereal can jump-start weight loss. When 60 people had high-fiber oatmeal for breakfast instead of low-fiber cornflakes, they ate 30 percent fewer calories at lunch, reported researchers from the New York Obesity Research Center at St. Luke's–Roosevelt Hospital. The appetite-control factor seems to be all that satisfying fiber, which helps you stay full.

Make a crunchy topping for fresh fruit. For dessert, serve oat-rich fruit crisps and cobblers. Just watch the butter content. It's better to use canola oil or a good-for-you brand of margarine, such as Smart Balance, instead.

Thicken with oats. Use oat flour or even a sprinkle of dry oat bran to stews, casseroles, and soups as a fiber-rich thickener.

Buy a bag of quick-cooking barley. Add it to soups, use it instead of arborio rice in risotto, and serve it as a nutty, flavorful side dish. The possibilities are endless. Pearled, hulled, or quick cooking, all varieties of barley are rich in cholesterol-lowering soluble fiber as well as compounds called beta-glucans that the human body converts into blood sugar extremely slowly. There's new evidence that eating barley at breakfast can keep you feeling fuller and more satisfied at lunch and even at dinner, so that you have fewer cravings and can make healthier choices at those meals.

Best Foods for Soluble Fiber

For healthier blood sugar levels, aim to fit as many of these foods as possible into your daily diet.

GRAINS	BEANS AND PEAS	VEGETABLES	FRUIT
Serving size: ½ cup cooked	Serving size: ½ cup cooked	Serving size: ½ cup cooked	Serving size: one medium fruit, except where noted
Oats: 1 gram	**Black:** 2 grams	**Broccoli:** 1 gram	
Barley: 1 gram	**Kidney:** 3 grams	**Brussels sprouts:** 3 grams	**Apple:** 1 gram
	Lima: 3.5 grams	**Carrots:** 1 gram	**Pear:** 2 grams
	Navy: 2 grams		**Blackberries** (½ cup): 1 gram
	Northern: 1.5 grams		**Orange:** 2 grams
	Pinto: 2 grams		**Grapefruit:** 2 grams
	Chickpeas: 1 gram		**Prunes** (¼ cup): 1.5 grams
	Black-eyed peas: 1 gram		

GOAL 3

Eat three servings of fruit a day

SOME PEOPLE GET THE IMPRESSION that the natural sugar in fruit makes this sweet treat off-limits for people with diabetes, but that just isn't the case. In fact, a June 2021 study in *The Journal of Clinical Endocrinology & Metabolism* found that participants who ate 1.5 servings of fruit per day had a 36 percent lower risk of developing type 2 diabetes than their peers who consumed less than half a serving. You'll be doubling that amount for even greater risk reduction.

Fruit is mostly water and fiber, so the amount of fructose it contains is fairly small. Meanwhile, fruits have almost all the advantages that vegetables do. They're brimming with nutrients, they're low in fat, they're high in fiber, and they're relatively low in calories. What it means: This is one sweet treat you can probably eat, in moderation of course, without worrying that your blood sugar will soar. (Dried fruits, especially raisins and dates, are another story.)

With a few exceptions, you can forget any "rules" you've heard about not eating *particular* fruits due to their effect on blood sugar. Truth is, it's personal. We recommend following your doctor's advice about blood sugar testing after meals and snacks to see how particular foods affect your blood sugar. You may find that certain fruits raise it more than others, which will influence your choices.

What's in a Fruit Serving?

Sprinkle a good handful of blueberries on morning cereal and voila—you've just given yourself one of your three daily fruit servings. What exactly constitutes a serving?

■ 1 medium piece of fruit

■ ½ cup chopped, cooked, or canned fruit

■ ¾ cup (six ounces) of 100 percent juice

■ ¼ cup dried fruit

STEP ONE

Start the Day with Fruit

Most of us don't eat vegetables at breakfast, so a piece of fruit is the perfect way to get fiber and important nutrients first thing in the morning. Here's how to add fruit to your break-of-day routine.

Make it a rule: Every breakfast includes a piece of fruit. Cantaloupe, an orange, berries—all are perfect with whole-wheat toast, cereal, or an egg. Or try sliced banana on wheat toast with a tablespoon of peanut butter or sliced apple with almond butter on a toasted whole-wheat English muffin.

Concoct a quick "baked" apple. Wash and chop an apple (leave the skin on for more fiber and nutrients), pile in a small bowl, sprinkle with cinnamon and cover with a microwave-safe paper towel. Microwave until soft, about 4 minutes. Enjoy with yogurt and oat bran sprinkles, or serve over oatmeal for a tummy-warming start on a cold morning.

Shred (yes, shred!) fresh fruit over yogurt. Choose plain, nonfat yogurt and dress it up with grated fresh fruit such as apples or pears (use the side of the box grater with the biggest holes for best results). Top with all-bran cereal for a fancy breakfast parfait.

Every Monday, start your week with a fruit smoothie. Add ½ cup fresh fruit, ½ cup plain nonfat yogurt, and one cup ice to a blender and liquefy. That's a serving of fruit before 8 a.m.!

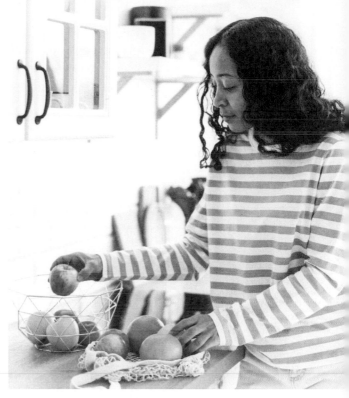

Whole fruit is almost always a good snack choice—far better than anything (except nuts) that you'd get from a bag.

STEP TWO
Make Fruit Ultra-Convenient for Snacking

Whole fruit is almost always a good snack choice—far better for your blood sugar and your waistline than anything (with the exception of nuts) that you'd get from a bag or a vending machine. Here's how to keep fruit ready at snack time—any time, any place.

Keep a fruit bowl filled wherever you spend the most time. This could be at work, near your home computer, or even in the television room. Keep it filled at all times with fruit such as bananas, oranges, apples, grapes, or plums. Most fruit is fine left at room temperature for three or four days. But if it's out and staring at you, it's not likely to last that long.

Bring fruit with you anytime you plan on driving for more than an hour. Once you are on the highway and cruising along, an apple or a nectarine tastes great and helps break the tedium. (Don't forget the napkins!)

Make a natural ice pop. Freeze banana slices or grapes for a delightfully refreshing cold summer treat.

Tuck an apple in your pocket whenever you go for long walks. It will be your reward for getting to the midpoint of your walk.

Keep cut-up melon in a clear container at the front of the fridge. Use as a first course before dinner; mix with low-fat cottage cheese for breakfast; have a small bowl for a snack; even consider pureeing for a quick sauce over fish.

Have "nice cream" instead of ice cream. Keep frozen, sliced bananas in your freezer. Then, when a hankering for sweets hits, pull some out, drop them in a blender, along with a dollop of peanut butter and a couple tablespoons of milk. Blend until it takes on the consistency of soft serve.

STEP THREE
Have Fruit at Lunch or Dinner Every Day

Fruit's a natural for snacking, and that apple in the afternoon counts as one of your three daily fruit servings. So did the fruit you had with breakfast.

Sugar Buster Quiz

Q: 100 percent juice or whole fruit?
A: Whole fruit

Many of the nutrients and a lot of the fiber found in the skin, flesh, and seeds of fruit are eliminated during juicing, and the calories and blood sugar–raising carbs are concentrated in juice, so you get more than you would if you ate the fruit.

That's Easy!

When you drink fruit juice, use a real juice glass, the kind your grandmother had. It holds just four or six ounces—a right-sized serving.

How to fit in one more serving? Plan on having some fruit at lunch, dinner, or both.

Sweeten your sandwich and add crunch. Add diced kiwi, sliced grapes, or chopped apple to chicken, tuna, and turkey salads.

Throw pineapples or peaches on the barbecue. Brush thick slices of pineapple or peaches with a little olive oil so they don't stick, then grill. Heat brings out the natural sweetness in the fruit.

Mix fruits in with your salad. Some cut-up strawberries, a diced apple, a small handful of grapes, or some sliced kiwi all make great additions to the typical tossed salad.

Top chicken or fish with fruit salsa. Make your own fruit-based salsas with pineapple, mango, or papayas. Mix with onions, ginger, a bit of garlic, some mint and/or cilantro, sprinkle on a few hot pepper flakes for fire, and chill.

Finish up with fruit. A slice of watermelon, a peach, a bowl of blueberries or raspberries topped with a dollop of yogurt—they're the perfect ending to a meal, and are so much healthier than cookies or cake.

Dress up fruit for a fancier dessert. A half-cup of strawberries drizzled with balsamic vinegar or soaked in white wine is a sweet, indulgent ending to your meal—and delivers 75 percent of your daily vitamin C requirement. (Recall that antioxidants help protect your body from the ravages of high blood sugar.) Or try roasted plums. Simply mix one teaspoon orange zest or ginger, ¼ cup orange juice, and one tablespoon pure maple syrup and simmer in a saucepan. Add two teaspoons of butter or trans-fat-free margarine and stir until melted. Place eight plum halves, cut side up, in a baking dish, top with the mixture, cover with foil, and bake 20 to 25 minutes at 400°F.

STEP FOUR
Go for Variety

Aim not only to eat more fruit but more *types* of fruit. If you only munch on apples or green grapes or strawberries, you're missing out on important, health-protecting nutrients that people with diabetes need—nutrients you'll get if you eat many different sorts of fruit. So that produce doesn't go bad, buy a combination of fruits that will keep for a while (such as apples and oranges), a small supply of more delicate fruits (such as berries and peaches) to eat in the first two days after you've gone shopping, and a back-up stash of frozen, no-sugar-added fruits such as berries and peaches in the freezer.

Start with these easy-to-find favorites. They are often tastiest and most affordable when purchased in season at a local farm stand or in the supermarket.

Apples. Researchers have discovered that women who eat at least one apple a day are 28 percent less likely to develop type 2 diabetes than those who don't eat apples. That's probably because apples, from tart Granny Smiths to sweet, juicy Pink Ladies, are loaded with soluble fiber—number one for blunting blood sugar swings. A medium apple dishes up an impressive two grams of fiber, mostly pectin, which is also known for its ability to lower cholesterol. Looking to trim your tummy? (News flash: Belly fat is bad for blood sugar.) Try eating three small apples a day.

Berries. From ruby red strawberries to midnight-blue blueberries, berries are candy for your taste buds—and powerful blood sugar controllers. Their sweetness is deceptive. Fructose, the natural sugar found in most fruits, is sweeter than what's in your sugar bowl (sucrose), so it takes much less, with fewer calories, to get that sweet taste. Berries are full of fiber, disease-fighting antioxidants, and red-blue natural plant compounds called anthocyanins that may help keep your blood sugar in check. Scientists believe anthocyanins, also found in cherries, may help lower blood sugar by boosting insulin production.

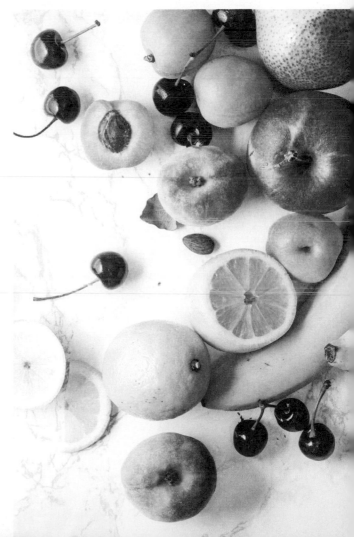

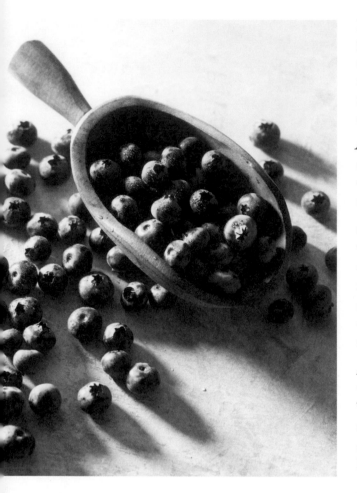

Be adventurous. Every month, buy one fruit you've never tried. Look no further than your local supermarket. Today's produce section is definitely not your grandmother's fruit stand. Here are some tips on what some of these unfamiliar fruits are and how to enjoy them.

Asian pear. Also called an Oriental, Chinese, salad, or apple pear, this firm pear is meant to be eaten immediately—when it's still hard. It's sweet, crunchy, and amazingly juicy.

Guava. It's sweet and fragrant with bright pink, white, yellow, or red flesh. Buy when it is just soft enough to press, and refrigerate for up to a week in a plastic or paper bag. To use, cut in half and scoop out the flesh for salads, or peel and slice. Try cooking and pureeing slightly under-ripe guava as a sauce for meat or fish.

Kiwi. This fruit never took off until they changed the name from Chinese gooseberry to kiwifruit. With a flavor that's a cross between strawberries and melon, kiwis are ready to eat when they're slightly soft to the touch. Peel and chop, or cut in half and scoop out the flesh with a spoon.

Lychee. Once, lychee trees were found only in southern China, but the popularity of this tropical fruit has caused its spread (it is now widely raised in Florida). The lychee fruit is about 1½ inches in size, oval, with a bumpy red skin. Peel off the inedible skin and you get a white, translucent flesh similar to a grape, but sweeter, surrounding a cherry-like pit. Eat 'em like large grapes. They're available only for a few months a year, but buy a pound next spring and discover why some call lychees the king of fruits.

Mango. This is one of the most commonly eaten fruits in the world, along with bananas. The flavor is a combination of peach and pineapple, but spic-

Peaches, plums, and apricots. These make perfect low-calorie snacks or sweet additions to entrées and desserts. They're easy on your blood sugar because, like most fruits, they have a high water content, plus a stash of blood sugar–taming, cholesterol-busting soluble fiber. Peaches boast the most fiber of the three. Apricots, which are close cousins to peaches, are richest in beta-carotene, linked with protection from heart disease and cancer. Plums are chock-full of several disease-fighting antioxidants, and dried plums outrank more than 20 other popular fruits and vegetables in antioxidant power.

ier and more fragrant (it is sometimes called the tropical peach).

Papaya. With soft, juicy, and silky-smooth flesh, papaya has a delicate, sweet flavor. The center of the papaya is filled with small, round, black, peppery-tasting seeds, which can be eaten but usually aren't. Peel, then slice into wedges or cut into chunks, or slice in half, remove seeds, and scoop out the flesh with a spoon. Unripe papayas can be peeled, seeded, and cooked as a vegetable, and you can grind the seeds like pepper for adding to sauces or salads.

Passion fruit. Passion fruit has golden flesh with tiny, edible black seeds and a sweet-tart taste. When ripe, it has wrinkled, dimpled, deep purple

Power Fruits

Of the hundreds of fruits out there, which ones give you the biggest nutritional bang for your buck? We bet on the ones with the most antioxidant power. Antioxidants neutralize free radicals—destructive molecules that damage cells. People with diabetes may have more free-radical damage than people without diabetes, raising risk for heart disease and other health problems. Which fruits pack the greatest antioxidant punch? The good people at the USDA figured it out. Here are the top 10.

1. Blueberries
2. Cranberries
3. Blackberries
4. Prunes
5. Raspberries
6. Strawberries
7. Red delicious apples
8. Granny Smith apples
9. Sweet cherries
10. Plums

Sugar Buster Quiz

Q: Fresh peach or canned peaches?
A: Fresh peach

Fruit you bite into wins hands-down over fruit you spoon from a can. A peach contains only 35 calories, whereas a cup of peaches canned in heavy syrup has 190. If you buy canned, go for peaches packed in their own juice (110 calories per cup).

or dark golden skin. To serve, cut in half and scoop out the pulp with a spoon.

Persimmon. Delicate in flavor and firm in texture, persimmons can be eaten like an apple, sliced and peeled, and are great in salads.

Pomegranate. It's the seeds of this crimson fall fruit that you eat. Each tiny, edible seed is surrounded by translucent, brilliant red pulp that has a sparkling sweet-tart flavor. Choose fruit that feels heavy for its size with bright color and blemish-free skin. They can be refrigerated up to a month, while the seeds can be frozen for three months. To serve, cut the fruit in half and pry out the seeds. Use them to top ice cream, sprinkle into salads, or simply eat as a snack.

Star fruit. Although they look exotic, most star fruits today come from south Florida. Slice them crosswise for perfect five-pointed star-shaped sections as a garnish or for fruit salads. Star fruit's flavor combines the best of plums, pineapples, and lemons.

GOAL 4

Include lean protein at every meal

WANT TO CONTROL YOUR BLOOD SUGAR and your weight? Get enough protein in your diet. Studies prove that protein helps keep hunger at bay between meals, and if you're trying to lose weight, taking in enough protein will also help your body hold on to its calorie-burning muscle tissue while you drop pounds.

But the benefits don't end there. Unlike carbohydrates, protein has little or no effect on your blood sugar. Eat a grilled chicken breast or a hardboiled egg and your levels will barely budge. It stands to reason, then, that if you substitute calories from protein for some of the calories you get from carbohydrates, your meals will have less impact on your blood sugar. And because your body breaks down protein slowly, including some turkey or beans with your pasta means that it will take longer for your body to digest the whole meal, resulting in a slower, gentler rise in blood sugar.

Just how important protein is for blood sugar control emerged from a fascinating study. Researchers at the University of Minnesota tested two diets, one high in protein and one with only half as much. The fat content was the same in both diets, but the carbohydrate content varied—volunteers ate fewer carbs on the high-protein diet, more carbs on the low-protein program. In the group that followed the high-protein diet, blood sugar levels were reduced by as much as if the participants had taken pills prescribed to lower blood sugar.

Does that mean that you should sit down to a 12-ounce T-bone steak or fried chicken tonight? No. Fatty cuts of beef, some cuts of pork, bacon, and many lunch meats pack lots of heart-threatening saturated fat, which raises levels of "bad" cholesterol. This "bad" fat has also been linked with increased insulin resistance, which contributes to higher blood sugar levels.

On the Eat plan, it's important to focus on lean protein foods, so that you get the blood sugar and

That's Easy! ◀

Put meat and poultry in the freezer for 20 minutes before you get to work trimming away excess fat. This will firm it up for easier cutting (the meat will become harder than the fat, making a closer "shave" possible) and make marbled fat more visible so you can locate and remove it.

weight-loss benefits of this important macronutrient without the health risks. The leanest proteins, of course, are plant-based ones, especially beans and legumes. And with some research showing an association between eating red meat and markers of insulin resistance, you may choose to follow a vegetarian, vegan, or plant-forward diet. If you do, rest assured that you absolutely *can* get enough protein without eating meat or dairy. If you're not quite ready to give up meat, poultry, or seafood, though, these steps can help you enjoy these foods healthfully.

STEP ONE

Have Lean Meat Up to Twice a Week

Yes, beef can still be for dinner—or, more accurately, *part* of *some* dinners if you choose. Here's how to get the leanest, most flavorful red meats on one-quarter of your plate.

Pair beef strips with veggies. Stir-fry strips of beef with lots of veggies for an easy way to have your beef and get your vegetables, too. Or throw together fajitas made with flank steak and generous amounts of bell peppers and onions for a quick weeknight meal. Or for a refreshingly delicious Asian-inspired salad, toss hot grilled beef with crisp lettuce, lime juice, and chopped onion.

Remake meat loaf. Create healthier meat loaf by combining finely chopped spinach and onions and grated carrots with extra-lean ground beef. Use oats as a binder.

Turn up the tenderness. Make any cut of beef a standout by marinating it in balsamic vinegar, olive oil, basil, Dijon mustard, and garlic. Or use any marinade that contains vinegar, wine, or

citrus juice. The acid softens the tissues of the meat, making it tenderer.

When company comes, serve up roast beef tenderloin. Don't forget to serve a salad beforehand and at least one veggie side dish.

Use half the beef; get all the flavor. In chili, tacos, spaghetti sauce, and casseroles that call for ground beef, use half extra-lean ground beef and

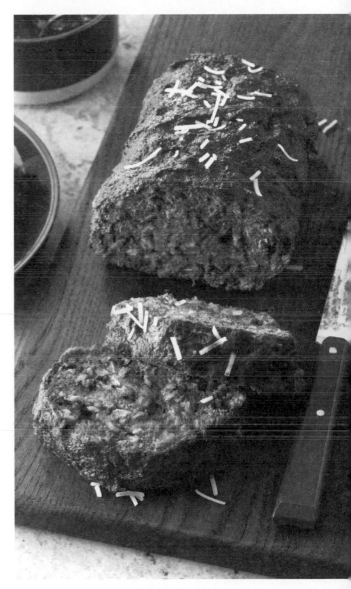

"Skinny" Beef

The following have 10 grams or less of total fat and 4.5 grams or less of saturated fat per serving. We've ranked them from the leanest to the least lean.

- ▶ Eye round roast
- ▶ Top round roast
- ▶ Mock tender steak
- ▶ Bottom round roast
- ▶ Top sirloin steak
- ▶ Round tip roast
- ▶ 95-percent lean ground beef
- ▶ Flat half of brisket
- ▶ Shank crosscuts
- ▶ Chuck shoulder roast
- ▶ Arm pot roast
- ▶ Shoulder steak
- ▶ Top loin steak (such as strip or New York steak)
- ▶ Flank steak
- ▶ Rib-eye steak
- ▶ Rib steak
- ▶ Tri-tip roast
- ▶ Tenderloin steak
- ▶ T-bone steak

half ground, skinless turkey, chicken breast, or even mushroom. You'll cut the fat content but still get the assertive, satisfying flavor of beef.

Take another look at pork. Pork loin is a very lean and affordable cut of meat that's flavorful and satisfying, such as beef. Among its charms: It cooks quickly in the oven or on the grill and tastes great with a wide variety of marinades and spices (we love garlic and oregano or low-sodium soy sauce and grated fresh ginger). Pork loin's perfect when company's coming for dinner. Or throw a couple of chops on the grill (try garlic-lime marinade or a rub made of chili and garlic powders).

STEP TWO

Turn to Chicken

Chicken and turkey can be high-fat disasters or perfect *Reverse Diabetes* fare. It all depends on the cut and how it's prepared. Breast meat is lower in fat than dark meat such as thighs and drumsticks. And in fact, a three-ounce serving of skinless chicken breast has 95 percent less saturated fat—the stuff that clogs arteries and blunts insulin sensitivity— than an equal serving of beef tenderloin. It also has 40 percent fewer calories, making it a practically perfect protein food. Just remember that even breast meat loses its health appeal when it's fried (especially in the oils used at many fast-food joints, which essentially turn chicken into a heart attack in a bucket). Most of the fat lies in the skin (though it is mostly unsaturated fat, so you don't need to be overly concerned about eating it).

Fortunately, lean poultry is incredibly versatile, as well as convenient. Here are easy ways to take advantage.

Enjoy a fast dinner of supermarket rotisserie chicken. Instead of the fast-food drive-through tonight, run into the supermarket for a bag of salad greens and a rotisserie chicken. At home, enjoy a big salad and a slice of breast meat. To keep it lean, skip the skin and don't eat the greasy drippings.

Order turkey or chicken breast at the deli counter. Roll up a few slices and add to salads to pump up their protein content, or eat them in sandwiches on whole-wheat bread topped with mustard, tomato, and plenty of lettuce or even baby spinach. Have two slices or 1.5 ounces per sandwich.

Roast some turkey even when it's not Thanksgiving. Turkey breast is actually lower in fat and cholesterol and higher in protein than chicken breast. You can now buy just the turkey breast in many grocery stores.

Try this instead of fried chicken. Brush boneless, skinless chicken thighs with olive oil and sprinkle with rosemary, salt, and pepper. Bake or grill until juices run clear, about 45 minutes. Chill overnight—this is great lunch or picnic fare. For another option that's just as finger-lickin' messy as the real thing, mix the juice of one lemon with one tablespoon Dijon mustard, ¼ cup honey, a pinch of curry powder, and a pinch of salt. Roll skinless chicken drumsticks in the mixture to coat well and bake until done, 45-60 minutes.

Use ground chicken or turkey breast in place of ground beef. Choose ground *breast* meat most often; that's the leanest pick. Ground chicken and turkey makes good burgers and tastes great in meat loaf, meatballs, chili, tacos, lasagna, and many other dishes.

STEP THREE
Have Fish Twice a Week

The fattiest protein on your plate should be oily cold-water fish such as salmon and mackerel (and to a lesser extent, tuna and other fish). These fish contain diabetes-fighting, heart-protecting omega-3 fatty acids—a fat you almost certainly need to get more of into your diet. A study at the Harvard School of Public Health found that women with diabetes who ate fish just once a week had a 40 percent lower risk of dying from heart disease than did women with diabetes who ate fish less than once a month.

The fats in fish do even more than guard against heart disease. They also cool chronic inflammation in the body, a major contributor to numerous chronic diseases, including insulin resistance and diabetes. Inflammation may even play a role in brain diseases such as Alzheimer's as well as certain cancers.

That's Easy!

Keep chicken tenderloins in the freezer for fast meals. Two tenderloins are about 3 ounces, a perfect portion. These skinless, boneless cuts thaw quickly in the fridge overnight or in a bowl of cold water (seal in a zip-close bag first).

Any fish is a great source of protein, and we encourage you to eat it twice a week when you might otherwise have chicken or beef. Shellfish counts, too, so go ahead and indulge in grilled shrimp, lobster, and mussels. They don't contain as much omega-3s as salmon, but they're still low in saturated fat and calories and rich in protein. Worried about your cholesterol? You don't need to avoid shrimp. It does contain cholesterol, but for most of us, shrimp should still get the green light. In a definitive Rockefeller University study, eating large servings of shrimp every single day raised "bad" LDL cholesterol by 7 percent, but it also boosted "good" HDL cholesterol 12 percent—a net benefit.

Here's how to fit in two servings of fish or seafood a week.

Keep frozen fish fillets in the freezer. Vacuum-packed sole, cod, or salmon fillets are the next best thing to fresh. You'll have dinner on the table in a flash—even if you have to spend a few minutes defrosting it first—because fish is done before you know it, making it a perfect weeknight meal.

Fire up the grill. Almost any type of fish tastes fabulous grilled, especially salmon. Brush it with a little olive oil to keep it from sticking. Throw some zucchini strips on the grill, too, and you have a blood sugar–friendly meal. Or try wrapping trout in foil with lemon slices, dill, thyme, salt, and pepper, and bake. Serve over quinoa.

No-Worries Salmon

An analysis involving a handful of researchers from different institutions came to this bottom line: Whenever you can, choose wild Pacific salmon instead of farmed salmon, which is typically higher in several chemical contaminants. If you do buy farmed salmon, which has higher levels of omega-3s and is usually cheaper, opt for farmed salmon from Chile. It's the healthiest and safest by far.

No matter which fish you choose, you're better off eating than not eating it.

Don't overlook salmon in cans and pouches. This is usually wild salmon—same as the pricey, sometimes hard-to-find stuff from the fish counter. Use it to make salmon salad or salmon croquettes and use in quiches and pasta dishes.

Stuff a tomato with tuna or salmon salad. Make the tuna or salmon salad with low-fat mayonnaise or plain yogurt, hard-boiled eggs, chopped apples, celery, and onion. Serve with whole-wheat crackers.

Think sushi for supermarket takeout. Many larger supermarkets have their very own sushi chefs on staff. If you need a quick, prepackaged meal, this is the place to stop. Sushi delivers protein and is generally low in calories. Since some types of sushi—especially bluefin tuna—may be contaminated with mercury, it's best to limit sushi to once a week.

Order grilled salmon when you dine out. You'll avoid temptations packed with saturated fat (such as cream sauces and deep-fried goodies) and ensure that you get a serving of healthy omega-3 fatty acids.

Keep a bag of frozen shrimp in the freezer. Thaw them according to the package directions and you have the makings of a fast, high-protein meal or appetizer. Serve boiled shrimp with shrimp sauce as a party hors d'oeuvres. Leftovers? Chop some cooked shrimp and sprinkle over your salad to add low-fat protein. Use a lemony dressing. Or place a shrimp, small chunks of avocado and tomato, and a bit of salsa on a lettuce leaf. Roll it up and eat! In stir-fries, use shrimp instead of chicken or beef. Add in the last five minutes to avoid overcooking. Also try shrimp instead of beef in your tacos.

Have lobster for lower blood sugar. Indulge in this fancy feast—without the melted butter. The upper crust of the crustacean kingdom happens to be a particularly rich source of a little-known mineral called vanadium, which studies suggest enhances insulin's effect in the body, helping to keep an anchor on blood sugar.

STEP FOUR
Enjoy "Bean Cuisine" at Least Three Times a Week

From black beans to chickpeas, cannelini to kidney beans, these slow-digesting little nuggets are rich in soluble fiber—and therefore fantastic for your blood sugar. In a recent study, men and women who ate a meal that included about 6 ounces of chickpeas had 40 percent lower blood sugar an hour after eating than those who ate an equal amount of white bread with jam.

The fiber in beans leads to a slow, steady blood sugar rise rather than a spike after a meal. Beans also pack loads of protein.

If you're trying to lose weight, eat beans! Not only are they incredibly filling, they also pack a heap of nutrition in a relatively low-calorie package. Better still, some of the starch in beans is a type called resistant starch that the body can't even digest, so the calories don't count. Beans are also full of folate, a B vitamin that may help reduce some of the nasty consequences of diabetes by helping to keep arteries clean.

The only downside for beans is the sodium content of canned beans. Choose reduced-sodium or no-salt-added beans and cut sodium by up to half by rinsing and draining them before using. Here are a handful of great ways to enjoy beans.

Put them on a bed of salad greens. Add chickpeas or kidney beans to a salad for a filling fix of protein. They're delicious with chopped red pepper, corn, and tomatoes.

Pour canned beans into soup or chili. Experiment with different combinations of colors, sizes, and flavors. Red and black beans are more assertive; white beans, a little sweeter.

Serve edamame as a side dish. These young green soybeans are wonderful snacks. You can buy them frozen; just steam and serve. They're also a perfect addition to soups and salads. Soy has more protein, ounce for ounce, than beef and almost none of the saturated fat.

Spruce up tomato sauce. Add white beans or chickpeas to pasta sauce along with chunks of vegetables for a hearty pasta topping.

Give them a starring role at your next picnic. Make a tasty salad by combining black beans with red onions, tomato, lime juice, cilantro, and shredded spinach.

Use in place of beef in Mexican foods. Mash kidney beans or black beans and use them on tortillas instead of beef or refried beans.

Create a high-fiber dip. Serve bean dip or hummus with a whole-wheat pita cut into wedges.

Cook up hearty chili. Cook up a big pot of black bean chili on the weekend and freeze the leftovers. Go meatless, or use ground skinless turkey or chicken breast in place of ground beef to keep saturated fat content low.

Bake chickpeas for a terrific snack. Whether the beans are canned or cooked dried, drain and pat dry. Toss about two cups beans with one beaten egg white and a mix of spices. Go for cumin, chili powder, and cayenne pepper for a spicy treat or cinnamon, ground ginger, and nutmeg for a sweet snack. Bake, stirring occasionally, at 400°F until golden and crisp, about 15 minutes.

That's Easy!

To get more beans into your diet, invest in a multicooker (such as the Instant Pot brand). These fantastic inventions allow you to soak and cook dried beans (and a whole host of other foods) in dramatically less time. To cook beans, use two cups water for every one cup beans. Add a teaspoon each of olive oil, salt, and baking soda. Set your cooker for 30 to 45 minutes, depending on the bean. Release the pressure, rinse, and store until ready to use.

STEP FIVE

Don't Forget Eggs

Eggs have been much maligned in recent years but the fact is, they're an excellent and inexpensive source of protein, and the most nutritionally complete of all protein sources. One large hard-boiled egg has seven grams of protein to keep you full, and just two grams of saturated fat. In studies, people who ate eggs and toast for breakfast stayed fuller longer and ate significantly fewer calories for the rest of the day than people who had a bagel and cream cheese. Because they're all protein and fat, eggs have virtually no impact on your blood sugar, making them a much better breakfast choice than, say, a stack of white-flour pancakes.

Eggs do contain cholesterol, but dozens of studies show that it's saturated fat, not dietary cholesterol, that raises people's cholesterol the most. For people with elevated cholesterol or those who are especially sensitive to the cholesterol in foods, experts recommend eating no more than three or four egg yolks a week. Egg whites, which contain no cholesterol, don't count.

If you have an egg tray in your refrigerator door, ignore it. Eggs stay fresh best if you keep them in their original container, pointed ends down.

Keep hardboiled eggs in the fridge for a protein-rich snack. It's hard to find snack foods rich in protein, but a hardboiled egg is the perfect solution. It's portable, too—but you do have to keep it cold.

Serve a frittata for dinner. Think of it as Italian egg pie. You can add almost anything to your frittata, such as lean ham, diced tomato, spinach, and goat cheese. Use one to two cups of filling for every four or five eggs.

Dress up egg salad sandwiches. Add veggies such as grated carrots, chopped leeks, finely chopped shallots, red onion, pea shoots, or plain old lettuce. Mix with a combination of low-fat mayo and plain yogurt. Sprinkle in a classic "egg salad" herb such as tarragon or dill. Or throw in some canned tuna to up your fish quotient for the day.

Sugar Buster Quiz

Q: Greek yogurt or regular yogurt?
A: Greek

Greek yogurt contains more than twice as much protein per serving as does regular yogurt, clocking in at about 20 grams per six ounces. By the way, cottage cheese and Skyr (an Icelandic dairy product that's similar to yogurt) are just as protein packed as Greek yogurt. Make sure to choose low or nonfat varieties.

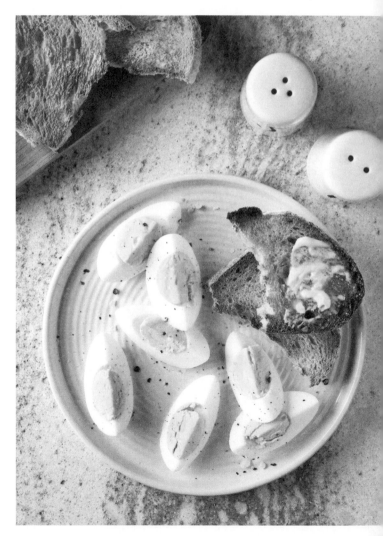

GOAL 5

Trade good fat for bad

THOUGH FATTY FOODS PACK more calories per gram than do carb or protein-rich foods, they also offer many benefits. Fat plays important roles in the body, helping to form cell membranes, distributing fat-soluble vitamins, and insulating the body against heat loss. And there's an upside to fat for diabetics: It slows the digestion process after a meal or snack, which means that glucose converted from the carbohydrates you've eaten enters the blood more gradually. As a result, fat should play a bigger role in your diet than you might assume—making up as much as 25 to 30 percent of total calories.

But not any old fat will do. As you've already seen, choosing the right fats can actually help your body process blood sugar better. Choosing the *wrong* fats contributes to insulin resistance, which makes blood sugar more difficult to control and raises your risk for heart disease, the number-one killer of people with diabetes. The fats to avoid? Saturated fats in fatty meats, poultry with the skin, and full-fat diary products such as whole milk, full-fat yogurt, and cheese. Also avoid the trans fats that still lurk in some margarines, commercial baked goods and snack foods, and processed and fast foods.

The right fats? These include monounsaturated fat found in nuts, nut butters, seeds, avocados, avocado oil, olive oil, and canola oil, as well as

That's Easy!

Grill time? Instead of burgers, here are some healthier options: salmon burgers, lentil burgers, veggie burgers, and ground chicken burgers. And instead of hot dogs, consider turkey kielbasa or apple chicken sausages.

omega-3 fatty acids, found in fatty fish, walnuts and hazelnuts, and to a lesser extent, flaxseed and flaxseed oil. Unlike saturated fat, which contributes to insulin resistance, these fats may even help reverse it.

The health benefits of these good fats are one reason that low-fat, high-carbohydrate diets are no longer seen as the healthiest eating strategy for people with diabetes. It's great knowing you can enjoy healthy fats without guilt or fear, and that you can harness these high-satisfaction, delicious foods to help you stay on track as you lose weight. We'll be honest. When it comes to fat—any fat—you still have to watch how much you eat. At nine calories per gram, even "good" fat can pack on the pounds. That's why you don't want to simply add good fats; you want to eat them *in place of* saturated fats and trans fats.

Here's how to enjoy good-fat foods without overindulging.

STEP ONE

Cut Way Back on "Bad" Fats

Your first step is to cut out, or significantly cut back on, the leading "bad fat" foods—see The Sat Fat Hit List below. Take special aim at full-fat cheese and fatty cuts of meat (think hamburgers, ribs, and bacon). If you avoid fast food and packaged treats (all too often made with oils full of saturated fat) and cook most of your meals at home, this shouldn't be all that hard to do, once you commit to doing it. Pick one food this week to cut back on, then next week, pick another. Don't worry—your meals will still taste great!

In Goal #4, you discovered smart ways to include lean meat and poultry in your meals. Now follow these additional tips to remove even more saturated and trans fats from your diet. Then read on for clever and flavorful ways to fill the gap with healthy good fats.

Slash saturated fat in meats. Follow all of our advice in Goal #4 to reduce saturated fat in the meats you eat. Choose leaner cuts of beef, remove the skin on chicken or turkey, and switch to ground skinless poultry instead of ground beef. Saturated fat from meats and poultry is a major source of this killer fat in the American diet.

Switch to nonfat milk. The fat in milk is the number three source of saturated fat in our diets, so it's time to go nonfat. You can even find fat-free half-and-half for your coffee. If you don't like the taste of nonfat milk, we have two suggestions. First, try ultra-pasteurized nonfat milk, which is thicker and creamier than regular nonfat milk. Or keep two cartons of milk in your fridge: one that's 2 percent and one that's nonfat. Blend them together, progressively adding more nonfat milk as you get used to it. You may also want to try a plant-based milk; just beware of brands with added sugars.

Say "cheese," only smarter. As a calcium-rich protein food, cheese has a (small) place in your diet. Unfortunately, most cheese is high in saturated fat. That means you'll want to use it sparingly. Make a little go a longer way by choosing a strong-flavored type such as Parmesan, Romano, or feta; you'll be able to use less and still get the taste you want. Also, look to lower-fat cheeses when possible. These include part-skim mozzarella, feta, and soft goat cheese.

Retire the fryer. Put away the fry bucket. Broiling, grilling, baking, and sautéing in avocado or olive oil are far healthier ways to prepare meals. Or try an air fryer.

Chill out. When preparing soups or stocks, chill broth overnight and skim off congealed fat.

Swap smart fats for margarine and butter. Rather than margarine on toast, try smashed avocado. For a baked potato, try nonfat Greek yogurt in place of both the margarine and the sour cream.

The Sat Fat Hit List

Americans get more "bad" fats from these foods than from any others. Often, you can make substitutes: low-fat cheese for full-fat hard cheeses, lean beef for high-fat cuts or burgers, nonfat milk for whole milk, olive or canola oil for soybean-based vegetable oil, fruit sorbet for full-fat ice cream. What will you substitute today?

1. Cheese
2. Beef
3. Milk
4. Coconut or palm oil
5. Ice cream, sherbet, frozen yogurt
6. Cakes, cookies, quick breads, doughnuts
7. Butter
8. Shortening, lard, other animal fats

In baked goods, experiment with replacing some of the butter with mashed avocado, banana, Greek yogurt, peanut butter, or unsweetened applesauce.

Take advantage of nonstick cookware. Why use butter or margarine to keep food from adhering to frying pans when nonstick pans will work. If you want to coat the pan, use a dab of olive oil or a quick spritz of cooking spray.

STEP TWO
Choose Your Oil Carefully

Using olive or avocado oil instead of butter or other oils is important. Unlike butter, these oils contain mostly smart fats, which don't increase insulin resistance and may even help reverse it, helping your body steady its blood sugar. Why not corn oil? It's thought to promote low-grade inflammation in the body, which contributes to diabetes, heart disease, and other health problems.

Like all fats, olive oil also slows digestion so that the bread or pasta you eat it with takes longer to break down into blood sugar. In an Australian study that compared the effects of consuming olive oil, water, or a mixture of water and oil before a high-carb meal, researchers discovered that it took almost three times as long for study volunteers' stomachs to begin emptying—significantly delaying the subsequent rise in blood sugar—when they had the olive oil. Slower rises in blood sugar also equates to feeling full longer, which in turn equals weight loss!

Olive oil is like liquid gold because it contains an anti-inflammatory component so strong that researchers liken it to aspirin. This may be one reason that people who follow the Mediterranean diet—a traditional way of eating that emphasizes olive oil along with produce, whole grains, and lean meat—have such low rates of heart disease and diabetes, both of which are linked with inflammation. Here's how to make the most of these versatile oils.

What's the Healthiest Cooking Oil?

When choosing a cooking oil, you want to consider several factors.

Fat profile All cooking oils contain a blend of saturated, polyunsaturated, and monounsaturated fats—but some oils are richer in some of those fat categories than others. For example, coconut oil, butter, and lard are richest in saturated fats, whereas olive oil, avocado oil, and canola oil (also called rapeseed oil) are richest in monounsaturated fats.

A study of 617,119 men and women found that replacing butter and margarine with canola or olive oil resulted in fewer deaths from heart disease. In another study, people with type 2 diabetes who added canola or olive oil to their diet were able to reduce levels of inflammation.

Cost Generally, canola oil will affect your pocketbook much less than more expensive olive and avocado oils. High-oleic sunflower oil is also a less expensive option that is rich in good fats.

Flavor Certain dishes call for different flavor profiles. Mediterranean dishes often call for olive oil, for example.

Smoke point Extra virgin olive oil starts to break down when heated to high temperatures, whereas canola and avocado can withstand temperatures of 400 degrees or higher.

Bottom line The best oil for you will depend on many factors. You might decide to invest in an expensive bottle of extra virgin olive oil that you use sparingly in salads and for drizzling. For roasting and other high-heat cooking, you might opt for avocado (if money is not an issue for you) or canola (if you're on a tight budget).

Dress your salads with the good stuff. Spring for a very nice extra-virgin olive oil for salad dressings. You'll taste the difference, and your salad will be that much more satisfying.

Cook with olive oil in place of butter or margarine. Great cooks use olive oil in just about everything. Use it whenever you can in place of other vegetable oils, margarine, or butter. (Use ¾ teaspoon olive oil in place of one teaspoon butter or margarine.) Note, however, that olive oil has a relatively low smoke point. Extra-virgin oil will start to break down—read burn—at about 375°F; virgin oil will start to burn at 420°F. When cooking at high temperatures, use avocado or canola oil instead.

Try a new topping for your potatoes. Try using a little olive oil mixed with roasted garlic instead of butter.

Dress up pasta with olive oil instead of butter or cheese. Add a teaspoonful to pasta, chopped tomatoes, crumbled feta cheese, chopped fresh basil, and capers for a fast and oh-so-simple supper.

Cholesterol-Friendly Margarine

One reason to limit your use of butter or margarine made with hydrogenated oil is that the kinds of fats they contain raise your cholesterol—definitely a bad thing if you have diabetes. But there is a way to have margarine and lower your cholesterol. Spreads such as Benecol and Take Control contain additives called sterols or stanols, plant chemicals that block the absorption of dietary cholesterol. Studies find that using a total of one to two tablespoons of this type of spread a day can cut cholesterol by as much as 10 percent.

STEP THREE

Have a Small Serving of Nuts or Seeds Five Times a Week

Thanks to their mix of good fat, fiber, and protein, nuts and seeds are "slow-burning" foods that are friendly to your blood sugar. In fact, Harvard researchers discovered that women who regularly ate nuts (about a handful five times a week) were 20 percent less likely to develop type 2 diabetes than those who didn't eat them as often. Believe it or not, people who include nuts in their diets also tend to weigh less.

Yes, nuts and seeds are high in fat, but it's about 85 percent good fat, the kind that may reduce insulin resistance. Good fats, of course, also improve heart health, even boosting levels of good HDL cholesterol. In studies, people who ate as few as five ounces of nuts a week as part of an overall heart-healthy diet lowered their risk of developing heart disease by 35 percent compared to those who ate nuts less than once a month. Here's how to fit nuts and seeds into your diet.

Use nuts to slow the digestion of carb-rich foods. Stir chopped walnuts or pecans into rice dishes. Mix pine nuts or chopped walnuts into pasta dishes along with olive oil, basil, and sun-dried tomatoes. Or create your own trail mix for snacking with dried fruit, high-fiber cereal, and your favorite nuts.

Give 'em a roast. Top off pumpkin, squash, or tomato soup with chopped roasted nuts. Or sprinkle your favorite chopped nuts and some dried cranberries on green salads. Roasting nuts brings out their flavor. Preheat the oven to 300°F. Place ½ cup of shelled nuts on a baking sheet in a single layer and roast for 7 to 10 minutes. Check near the end of the roasting time to make sure they don't burn.

Enjoy peanut butter sandwiches again. Peanut butter and other nut butters—such as almond or cashew butter—make delicious lunch-time sandwiches, especially if you spread them on coarse whole-grain bread and top with fruit instead of jelly. Banana's an obvious choice, but we also love the taste of strawberries, sliced apple, peaches, and pears on a nut-butter sandwich with a sprinkle of cinnamon or nutmeg for an added boost of flavor. Just be careful not to overdo it. One serving is two tablespoons, which is roughly the size of two thumbs.

Introduce yourself to flaxseed. Tiny, shiny, and brown, flaxseeds are a godsend to your blood sugar as well as your heart, so if you haven't tried them yet, it's time for a trip to the store. Flaxseed is rich in both protein and fiber (more than 2 grams per tablespoon of ground seeds). It's also a good source of magnesium, a mineral that's key to good blood sugar control because it helps cells use insulin. But what's really unique about these seeds is this: They're incredibly rich in an essential fatty acid called alpha linolenic acid, which the body uses to make the same type of omega-3 fatty acids you get from fish. Ground flaxseed spoils quickly, so buy whole seeds in bulk and grind as needed. (Warning: Eat them whole and they'll come out the same way they went in.) Whole seeds will last up to a year stored at room temperature. If you buy ground flaxseed, keep it in the fridge.

Sprinkle ground flax. Once you discover flax-seeds you'll find countless uses for them. They're great on hot or cold cereal, yogurt, or low-fat ice cream. You can add them to meat loaf, meatballs, burgers, and casseroles, or add a tablespoon or two to doughs and batters for pancakes, waffles, muffins, and breads. (Just keep an eye on baked goods in the oven; the flaxseed could make them brown quicker than usual.) Add them to cooked

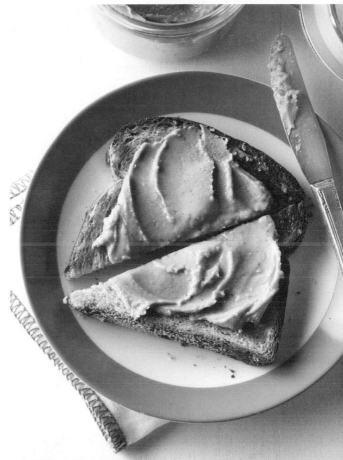

Thanks to their mix of good fat, fiber, and protein, nuts and seeds are friendly to your blood sugar.

fruit desserts such as baked apples or blueberry compote.

Add chia seeds. High in protein, omega-3 fatty acids, minerals and antioxideants, chia seeds are great in smoothies, salad dressings, and mixed into cereal or baked goods.

Discover the super-seeds. Pumpkin, and sunflower seeds (buy unsalted varieties) make great snacks along with a piece of fruit. They're also a tasty replacement for croutons on a salad or sprinkled lightly over steamed green beans or carrots.

STEP FOUR
Use Avocado Instead of Butter and Cheese

This rich, creamy fruit is loaded with fat—a whopping 25 to 30 grams each—but most of it good monounsaturated fat, the same fat you get in nuts and olive oil. Research suggests that diets rich in this type of fat may help keep blood sugar in check by slowing digestion after a meal. And unlike the saturated fats in butter and meat, monounsaturated fat won't increase insulin resistance. There is even some suggestion that eating more monounsaturated fat could help insulin-producing cells in your pancreas stay healthier. That means avoca-

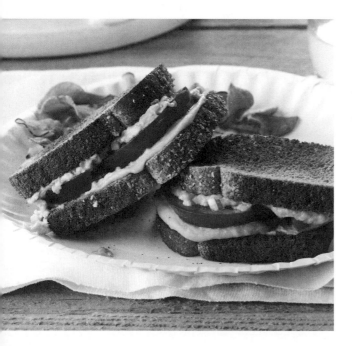

That's Easy!

To prevent a cut avocado from turning brown in the refrigerator, remove the seed and spray the flesh with cooking spray, then wrap in plastic. Use within three days. If avocados are ripening faster than you can eat them, mash them with ½ tablespoon lemon or lime juice per avocado. Place in an airtight container, cover, and freeze. Use within four months.

dos are great additions to your diet if you eat them in moderation.

Start with a ripe avocado. Hold the avocado in your hand and press it gently, then roll it to the other side and press again. If it gives just a bit but pressure doesn't leave a permanent dent (an indication that it's too ripe), it's ready to eat.

Eat it as a snack. Instead of a handful of pretzels—practically all carbs—or cheese, cut an avocado into five pieces and eat two of them, drizzled with lemon juice, for a satisfying 110-calorie snack.

Use avocado in place of cheese. Have a slice on your sandwich for 55 calories—half the 100 or so calories in an ounce of cheese. Or mash some avocado and spread it on in place of mayonnaise.

Add to salads. Use chunks or slices in place of cheese, or mash avocado and mix with lemon juice for a thick, dressing-like addition. Adding it to salads also increases your body's ability to absorb the good-for-you carotenoids, such as beta-carotene, in salad greens.

GOAL 6

Use the Plate Approach for perfect portions

NOW YOU'RE READY to get down to the nitty-gritty—putting the healthy, tasty foods you've read about in Goals #1 through #5 on your plate. Your assignment: Get a plate and set yourself a place at the table. Learning to fill it with perfect portions of fruit and vegetables, smart carbs, and protein is the key to successful blood sugar control, successful weight loss, and success at lowering your risk for diabetes complications.

The good news: Using the Plate Approach can make weighing and measuring food for portion control obsolete.

The Plate Approach rebalances your meals to give you the ideal proportions of vegetables, protein, and carbohydrates. Using the Plate Approach *automatically* cuts your calorie intake—the real goal of any weight-loss plan. It also ensures that you won't get too many carbohydrates at one sitting, with no need for you to keep a tally. Best of all, your plate will contain plenty of food, so you'll never feel deprived.

Complicated eating plans, such as the food exchange system that dietitians sometimes recommend for people with diabetes, are supposed to be effective because they make you track every-

thing you eat, theoretically leaving less to chance. But many people find the exchange system too confusing. The Plate Approach accomplishes the same objective (controlling portions and calories) in a simpler way—and it works.

In one study at Emory University School of Medicine in Atlanta, people who used a basic visual guide to make healthy choices lowered

Do You Need a Stricter Approach?

The Plate Approach automatically controls carbs and therefore helps regulate blood sugar. However, if you use insulin or you're having trouble controlling your blood sugar, you may need a stricter approach, such as carbohydrate counting, a system that helps you keep tight control on carb levels at every meal. Consult a registered dietitian who can customize a plan for you and refer to the carbohydrate counts starting on page 186. You can combine carb-counting with the Plate Approach to achieve better blood sugar control and to reach a healthy weight.

The Plate Approach
at a Glance

Using the Plate Approach, the number of calories you save by eating more vegetables and fewer fatty foods can be significant. See for yourself. Because the meal on the bottom also contains fewer starches, it should have much less of an impact on your blood sugar.

TYPICAL AMERICAN MEAL
Calories: 1,358

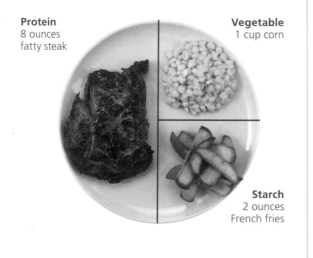

Protein
8 ounces
fatty steak

Vegetable
1 cup corn

Starch
2 ounces
French fries

PLATE APPROACH MEAL
Calories: 440

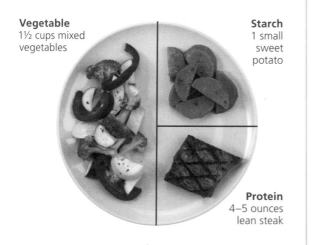

Vegetable
1½ cups mixed
vegetables

Starch
1 small
sweet
potato

Protein
4–5 ounces
lean steak

their blood sugar, cut calories, and lost weight just as successfully as those who took the trouble to follow a plan that used food exchanges. And in a Canadian study, people with diabetes who followed a similar Plate Approach lost more weight than those who got conventional weight-loss advice. And they kept using their Plate Approach even after the study ended.

The biggest change you'll likely see on your plate? That humble helping of vegetables in the typical American meat-and-potatoes dinner will become a hearty helping, shrinking the space left over for fatty meat and carbs—the major sources of calories, fat, and blood sugar-raising starches and sugars.

Use the three main elements of a typical meal—meat, carbs, and vegetables—as your starting point. When you dish them out, your plate in effect becomes divided into three sections. Of course, it's the size of the sections that matters. To picture how your plate should look on the Plate Approach, mentally divide it into left and right halves. Then imagine the right half split into two equal parts. Whenever you eat a meal, keep these sections in mind and fill them in the following way.

STEP ONE
Load the Left Half of Your Plate with Vegetables (and Fruit)

The entire left side of your plate is reserved for produce. This is where you'll put all of your vegetables as well as fruit. Choose anything you like except potatoes and corn.

There's no escaping it: To lose weight, you need to take in fewer calories than you burn. The Plate Approach's solution to cutting calories is remarkably simple: Eat more vegetables and less of everything else. In the Plate Approach, half the real estate on your plate is taken up by vegetables, which are naturally very low in calories, so there's less room for starches and calorie-dense meats.

Vegetables are low in calories yet high in volume because a lot of their weight comes from water. Such high-volume foods have the advantage of looking big, so they make your brain expect that you'll be satisfied by eating them. They also take up more room in your stomach, so they trigger a signal in your brain that makes you stop eating sooner. It's small wonder that researchers in weight-loss programs such as that at the University of Alabama in Birmingham find that when people eat lots of vegetables, their calorie consumption goes down—and they lose weight.

Still hungry? You can fill the biggest portion of your plate—the vegetable section—again and again. That's right, there's no limit on the amount of food you can eat from this part of the plate as long as you stop when you feel satisfied. On the right half of the plate, however, stick with one helping of carbohydrate and one helping of protein.

Almost all vegetables are inherently good for you, but beware of transforming low-calorie vegetables into high-calorie ones by frying them in oil or smothering them with toppings, such as cheese sauces, full-fat salad dressings, or butter.

> **Vegetables are low in calories yet high in volume because a lot of their weight comes from water.**

A word about breakfast: We're not going to ask you to fill half your plate with vegetables at this meal, since most of us don't eat vegetables in the morning (although if you're making an omelet, go ahead and pack it with as much produce as possible). Instead, substitute fruit, such as blueberries, strawberries, or bananas.

STEP TWO
Fill the Upper Right-Hand Side with Smart Carbs

Grain-based carbohydrates and starchy veggies such as potatoes belong in the upper right-hand side of your plate. This area is reserved for whole-grain pasta, brown rice, barley, noodles, potatoes,

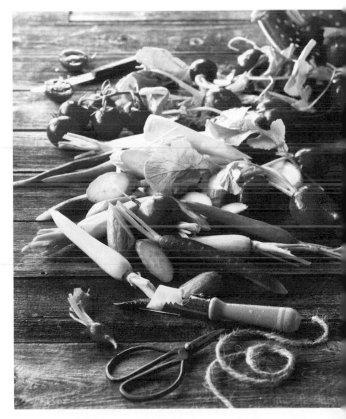

or corn. If you're serving starchy beans (legumes such as black beans, pinto beans, kidney beans, or chickpeas) as a side dish, you would put them here.

The benefit? When starches are limited to one-fourth of your plate, you've got automatic carb control, which translates into better blood sugar control.

You already know that carbs aren't dietary disasters and that having three servings of whole grains a day will enhance your health and your blood sugar if you have diabetes. But limiting portions is important with both starchy and grain-based carbs. First, they raise blood sugar. Second, some researchers now believe that eating too many carbohydrates makes weight control especially hard for people who are already heavy. The reason: Carbs break down easily into glucose, and with enough glucose on hand, the body never has to burn its fat stores for energy.

With the Plate Approach, you'll enjoy a generous yet safe and controlled amount of carbs—no more worries about overeating second helpings of rice or mashed potatoes, no more guilt.

STEP THREE
Put Lean Protein on the Bottom Right-Hand Side of Your Plate

Reserve one-fourth of your plate for satisfying, sugar-controlling protein foods. These include lean red meat, eggs, fish, chicken and turkey, as well as dairy products such as yogurt or cheese. If legumes are part of your entrée, put them here.

You've already learned that making sure you get protein at every meal is critical. Protein makes you feel full longer than carbohydrates do, and it doesn't raise blood sugar. So why not eat more

of it? We're glad you asked. The first reason, of course, is calories. Just about any protein food you eat has more calories than veggies do. The second reason is fat. As you know now, saturated fats directly impair the body's ability to react to insulin, the hormone that keeps blood sugar in check, and many protein foods contain these fats. Finally, if you fill up on protein at the expense of vegetables or whole grains, your body will be deprived of nutrients that are essential for good health.

STEP FOUR
Internalize the Plate Approach

Not every meal will fit precisely onto different segments of a plate the way we've suggested. For example, a stir-fry might have all the right elements—carbs (brown rice), lean protein (chicken strips), and lots of vegetables (carrots, broccoli, and pea pods)—but the ingredients are mixed together. That's OK. Once you get the basic idea of the Plate Approach down and get used to seeing how much food goes into each section of the plate, you won't need the divisions to guide you. As long as the bulk of the dish is vegetables, with smaller amounts of rice and poultry, a stir-fry is a perfect Plate Approach meal.

You may also have problems using the Plate Approach when you're out to dinner, eating a meal that isn't served on a dinner plate, or eating food that you didn't serve yourself. In these situations, having a sense of how a healthy portion looks will help you stay on track. See A Visual Guide to Portion Sizes on the opposite page.

A Visual Guide to Portion Sizes

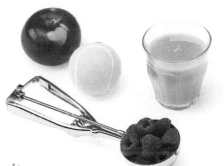

Fruit
A serving is:

One medium piece of fruit (the size of a tennis ball)

¾ cup fruit juice

½ cup chopped, cooked or canned fruit, or berries (the size of a large ice cream scoop)

Vegetables
A serving is:

¾ cup vegetable juice

½ cup nonleafy vegetables, cooked, chopped, or canned (the size of a large ice cream scoop)

One cup raw leafy vegetables (the size of a baseball)

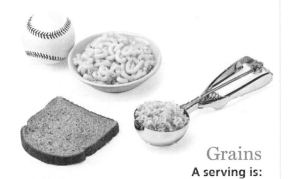

Meat, Poultry, Fish & Beans
A serving is:

Three ounces of cooked lean meat, poultry, or fish (the size of a deck of cards)

½ cup of cooked dry beans (the size of a large ice cream scoop)

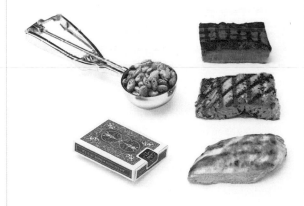

Grains
A serving is:

½ cup cereal, rice, bulgur, or barley (the size of a large ice cream scoop)

½ cup pasta (two servings equals the size of one baseball)

One slice of bread

GOAL 7

Plan your meals

HERE'S A FOOLPROOF WAY to ensure you don't follow Eat Goals #1 through #6: Wait until just before a meal to decide what to eat.

Without planning your meals and snacks ahead of time, mental fatigue and hunger can strongly lure you toward highly palatable, convenient options such as tater tots, delivery pizza, chips, sweets, fast food, and that dessert your coworker left on the table in the breakroom.

Another problem: Lack of planning means you may not always have healthy foods on hand. In other words, even if you were craving raw cauliflower, you're still out of luck.

Meal planning helps you to overcome the above issues—and you don't have to take our word for it. The NutriNet-Santé study of 40,554 participants found that meal planners were more likely to adhere to nutritional guidelines and had a lower odds of being overweight.

Use this five-step process to get in the habit.

STEP ONE
Decide What You Want to Make

Once a week, spend time thinking about what you want to eat for your meals and snacks during the week ahead. If planning all of your meals and snacks feels overwhelming, start with what feels most doable. Maybe you start by planning only your snacks. Once that feels like a snap, you might add breakfast, then lunch, and then dinner.

Another alternative: Rather than planning a full seven days worth of meals, you might plan just two or three days ahead of time. Once you have that down, plan four or five, then six or seven.

When figuring it what to eat, consider the following:

The Reverse Diabetes Plate. Use Plate Approach principles to guide your choices and portion sizes. For lunch and dinner, include some protein, a moderate portion of whole grains, and a hearty serving of veggies. For breakfast, it's OK to sub in fruit for your veggie portion, if needed. For snacks, aim for two of the three plate categories, such as a veggie and a protein or a protein and a smart carb.

See the 35 Reverse Diabetes Plate Ideas on page 78-79 for ideas.

Your calendar. Take a look at your week ahead so you can get a handle on how much time you can devote to each meal.

Are there any mornings when you need to roll out of bed and head straight to an appointment? If so, a grab-and-go breakfast (say, a couple of hard-

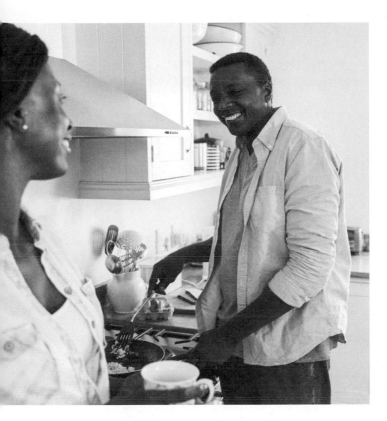

as casserole night, Tuesday as grilled fish night, and Wednesday as roasted chicken night. Include tried-and-true vegetable and whole-grain side dishes as well.

Similarly, perhaps you decide to automate breakfast, snacks, and/or lunch—choosing from just one, two, or three options rather than planning a completely new meal each day of the week.

What's currently stocked in your kitchen. Is there anything you want to use up before it's too late? If so, consider looking for recipes based on that ingredient.

A backup plan. Here's a life truism: Stuff goes wrong. In other words, despite your best plans, sometimes you forget to defrost that chicken. Or your work day goes sideways. Or you're just not in the mood for the meal you planned. That's when it helps to plan for an emergency meal, such as avocado toast with a fried egg.

Themes. Rotating through a series of themed meals can help you automate planning. Here are some themes to consider:

- Chicken night
- Slow or instant cooker night
- Taco night
- Casserole night
- Sheet pan meal night
- Breakfast-for-dinner night
- Leftover night
- Seafood night
- Stir-fry night
- Grain bowl night
- Burger night
- Soup and sandwich night
- Sandwich and salad night

Inspiration. Every once in a while, you may struggle to come up with ideas for what to eat. That's

boiled eggs and a store-bought container of sliced fruit) might be the way to go.

Similarly, will you need to pull off a speed dinner so you can shuttle kids or grandkids to activities? If so, leftovers, sandwiches, smoothies, or premade turkey burgers might come in handy. Or maybe you plan to put something in the slow cooker in the morning so it's ready by the time you come home.

Your capacity for cooking. No one expects you to come up with a new meal every night. The trick is to find 8 or 10 healthy meals you love (you may even want to keep a list on your refrigerator), then rotate them in. Start with three low-fuss, nutritious options that you can almost cook in your sleep. For example, you might designate Monday

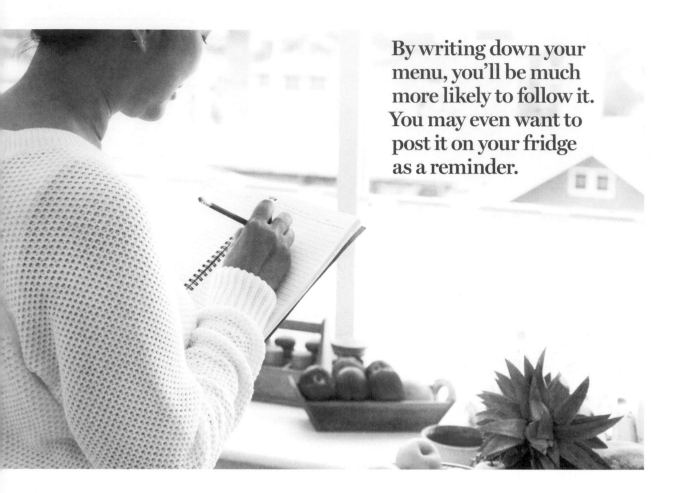

By writing down your menu, you'll be much more likely to follow it. You may even want to post it on your fridge as a reminder.

normal and expected. One way to overcome this problem: Continually inspire yourself by following cooks you like on social media, signing up for recipe newsletters, buying cookbooks, or subscribing to magazines.

STEP TWO
Make Your Plan a Little Better

Think of Step 1 as a free-form brainstorm.

Step 2 is where you look at your plan with a critical eye, asking yourself:

Can I make this a little bit healthier? In other words, can you add veggies to that soup recipe you found on the Internet? Can you swap whole grain pasta in for regular? Could that grilled cheese sandwich benefit from a little spinach and turkey, not to mention thin-sliced whole grain bread?

Can I make this a little bit easier? Maybe you decide to use parts of one night's dinner for the following night's meal, batch cook grains early in the week, or make complicated recipes on the weekends. Or perhaps you build meals from canned beans, rotisserie chicken, bagged lettuce mix, pre-chopped fruit and other convenience items.

STEP THREE

STEP THREE

Write Down Your Plan

We've provided a meal planner template on page 176; you can also find a downloadable version at thehealthy.com/reversediabetes/mealplanner.

By writing down your menu, you'll be much more likely to follow it. You may even want to post it on your fridge as a reminder.

Scan to find the planner online.

STEP FOUR

Create a Shopping List Based on Your Plan

With your plan in place, look at each recipe and meal idea. Go through your kitchen. Do you have everything you need? Add to the list what's missing, along with the amount you need.

This is also a great time to take a look at your pantry to see if you need to top off any staples such as olive oil, spices, or flour.

Once you have a list, combine items and reorder everything by area of the grocery store. Our grocery list template

Scan to find the list online.

on page 177 or thehealthy.com/reversediabetes/shoppinglist does this for you.

STEP FIVE

Shop and Cook

Once you have everything you need, just one task remains: get cooking. Save your menus from week to week so you can reuse them as desired.

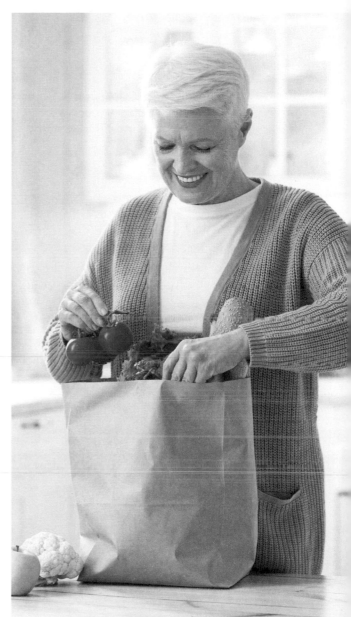

Think about how you can make your plan a little bit healthier and a little bit easier.

35 Reverse Diabetes Plate Ideas

Each suggested meal contains lean protein, veggies and/or fruit, smart carbs, and healthy fat. Each snack suggestion features food from at least one of those categories.

Breakfast Ideas

Hard-boiled eggs + sliced apple with peanut butter

Veggie omelet + one whole-grain English muffin

Roasted turkey and cheese roll up + sliced cucumbers + one orange

Greek yogurt mixed with berries, pumpkin seeds, and high-fiber cereal

Oatmeal cooked with chopped apple and mixed with Greek yogurt

Whole grain toast topped with mashed avocado and fried eggs + sliced banana

High-protein and/or high-fiber breakfast cereal with milk and fruit

Whole-grain English muffin sandwich with fried egg, sliced tomato, and spinach

Whole grain toast topped with peanut butter and banana

Lunch Ideas

Whole grain turkey, cheese, and sprouts sandwich + side salad

Leftover sliced pork tenderloin + brown rice + sliced bell pepper

Salad topped with grilled chicken, roasted sweet potato, and olive oil vinaigrette

Brown rice bowl: brown rice + cooked shrimp, salmon, or chicken + veggies of your choice + avocado

Bean salad: Black beans + corn + avocado + dressing (olive oil/lime juice)

Veggie wrap: Grind baby spinach with ricotta and Pamesan cheese and wrap in a whole-wheat tortilla. Serve with sliced fruit

Leftover chili made with beans and ground turkey + salad

Pita pizza: Whole grain pita topped with sliced broccoli, mozzarella, and tomato sauce. Serve with a salad.

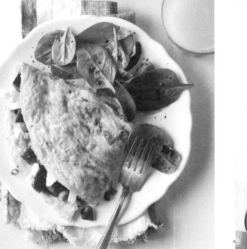

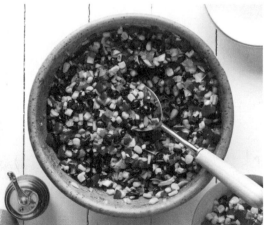

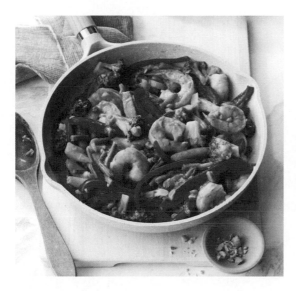

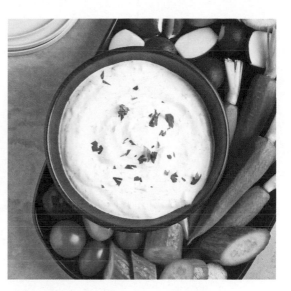

Dinner Ideas

Brown rice + roasted salmon and broccoli

Barley + baked chicken + salad

Whole grain pasta topped with chicken Parmesan and roasted zucchini

Turkey meatballs with linguine, tomato sauce, mushrooms, and cherry tomatoes

Stir-fry of shrimp and precut veggies, served over ½ cup brown rice or barley.

Barbecued chicken breast or tofu "steak" + steamed broccoli + strawberries + an ear of corn

Lasagna made with lots of vegetables, ground skinless chicken or turkey, whole-wheat noodles, and fat-free ricotta, served with a tossed salad.

Baked or grilled fish + sautéed spinach + steamed carrots + barley.

Steamed or stir-fried vegetables mixed with ½ cup whole-grain pasta, sliced chicken breast, and a dusting of Parmesan cheese. Serve with a tossed salad.

Pork tenderloin or a center-cut pork chop + steamed green beans with sliced almonds + one-half of a baked sweet potato

Whole grain vegetarian pinwheel: Smear whole grain tortilla with pureed beans. Top with baby spinach and slivered celery and carrots. Roll and then slice into bite-sized pieces.

Snack Ideas

Greek yogurt + berries

Greek yogurt + nuts/seeds

Celery stuffed with peanut butter

Veggies dipped in hummus or guacamole

Roast beef and cheese rolled with celery sticks

Sliced apple topped with peanut butter

Cucumbers, carrots and cherry tomatoes with yogurt-based dip

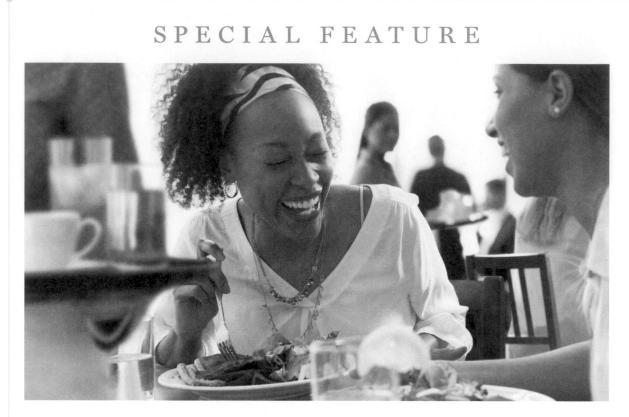

Dining Out Wisely

Who doesn't love dining out, whether it's breakfast at your favorite neighborhood diner, a quick lunch in a delicious deli, or a relaxing dinner? When you eat out, eat smart, following the same eating goals you use at home. Avoid oversized portions, excess fat, and an overload of refined carbohydrates, (The bread basket! The mountain of pasta! The desserts!) and the only price you'll pay will be your check, not your health.

Restaurants are in the business of making you feel like a VIP. All the low lighting, soft music, and mouthwatering scents drifting from the kitchen are designed to make you stay longer. Add an indulgent wait staff and

a cocktail or glass of wine before your meal, and you're set up to adopt a devil-may-care attitude toward what you order and how much of it you eat. The best way to avoid overindulging is to walk through the door prepared.

Eat Smart While Eating Out

These strategies tip the odds in your favor for getting a blood sugar-friendly meal in any restaurant.

Choose your restaurant with care. Make the challenge of eating out easier by being smart about what kinds of restaurants you patronize.

Avoid the temptation of all-you-can-eat places or buffet-style restaurants, where portions are hard to control. Avoid places known for enormous portions, such as many chains and most steak houses. And you probably won't find a lot of *Reverse Diabetes* foods on the menu at eateries that specialize in deep-frying an entire breaded onion. Enjoy a meal at one of these on your birthday, sure, but don't do it on a regular basis.

Check out the website before you go. Many restaurants post calorie counts and other nutritional information for their dishes online. Review these ahead of time to decide what your best choices might be.

Make friends with the server. Once you're in the right kind of restaurant, get ready to get friendly with the server. Ask them to hold the bread basket. Inquire about how a dish you're considering is prepared, and find out how big the portions are. At the same time, ask for a glass of water. Remember to drink plenty of water with your meal.

Order creatively. When you order, be bold: Order soup, salad, and an appetizer (not fried) for your meal rather than an entrée. Split an entrée and share a side order of vegetables to get more veggies into your meal and cut calories. If a main dish comes with a potato, ask if you can get an extra vegetable instead. (Especially if you're a regular customer, you're likely to get your way.) If you plan to order dessert, plan to share it, too. The best situation is when you get to know a restaurant's regular fare, including how big the portions are, and use that knowledge to outsmart the menu.

Draw the line. Ask whether the kitchen can prepare half portions. Many restaurants are more than willing to do so. Some even offer half portions on the menu. If the dish you order turns out to be too big, ask the servernright then and there to divide the portion and set half aside for you to take home. Don't wait until you've started to nibble, and don't depend on your willpower to eat only half of what's in front of you. If you know in advance that the entrées at a particular restaurant are outsized, ask for a half portion as the meal and request that the other half be brought at the end in a takeout container.

Be colorful. Meat and creamy sauces are usually brown, right? Where do most dishes get their brightest colors? From vegetables and fruit, of course. Choose the most colorful dishes on the menu, and chances are you'll order the healthiest, lowest-calorie selections. Spicy red salsas, deep purple beets, green salads, yellow corn, bright orange and yellow sweet peppers turn your plate into a rainbow of colors. As long as vegetables arrive without added fat, they're yours to eat to your heart's (and your blood sugar's) content.

Dip into the sauce. Ordering salad dressing on the side and drizzling it on sparingly is one of the oldest healthy-eating tricks. Remember that you can order other sauces on the side, too, from gravy to guacamole. Give yourself no more than a tablespoon. And put your fork to good use.

Steer clear of anything breaded, crispy, creamy, or buttery. Choose grilled, baked, steamed, or broiled foods instead. When ordering soups and sauces, stick with those that are broth-based or tomato-based.

Stick to one drink—and have it with your meal. Wine, beer, and liquor add calories to your meal and may encourage overeating.

continued >>>

Eating Out Italian

A single slice of pizza with vegetables is a fine choice, especially if it's made with a whole-wheat or thin crust. A cup of pasta with marinara sauce is all right, too. The problem is, few of us stop there.

Ironically, southern Italian food, prepared the traditional way, is among the healthiest in the world. Unfortunately, Italian restaurants are often parlors for the presentation of huge mounds of overcooked pasta and pizza. And even before these arrive, you'll have ample opportunity to eat bread. So unless you want to overload on carbs and send your blood sugar for a wild post-meal ride, tread carefully. Here's how.

If you want pasta, order a dish from the appetizer section of the menu, or share. That's the traditional way—a small first course of pasta followed by simple grilled meat, poultry, or fish and a side of sautéed greens. When your plate arrives, use your fist to designate the size of your serving. Move the overflow to the side of your plate—and look forward to having it as leftovers. Top it with lots of veggies, if possible, or a light tomato- or wine-based sauce.

If it's on the menu, order simple grilled beef, veal, pork, chicken, fish, or shellfish. Add a side order of sautéed spinach or broccoli rabe (a slightly bitter Italian version of broccoli). Finish with a mixed green salad with vinaigrette dressing.

For dessert, ask for fresh berries or fruit ice, if it's available, or a small plate of cookies to share. Stay away from the custards and cheesecake, the cannoli and the tiramisu.

WHAT TO ORDER

■ Appetizers/Sides

Minestrone soup; pasta e fagioli (fagioli means "beans"); green salad; grilled or marinated vegetables; broiled shrimp (no butter); steamed mussels.

■ Entrées

Pasta with marinara or Bolognese sauce; pasta with red clam sauce; chicken cacciatore; chicken or veal marsala; grilled fish; mixed grill; thin-crust cheese or vegetable pizza; Caprese salad; fruita de mare.

WHAT NOT TO ORDER

■ Appetizers/Sides

Garlic bread; fried mozzarella sticks; antipasto (it's mostly high-fat cheese and high-fat meat); stuffed mushrooms (usually high in fat).

■ Entrées

Pasta with Alfredo (cheese) sauce; penne alla vodka; shrimp scampi (rich in butter or oil); pasta primavera (usually made with cream); fried calamari or anything else that's fried; eggplant parmigiana (eggplant is a sponge for oil); anything stuffed.

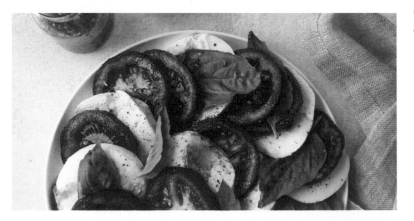

Eating Out Mexican

Ordering from a fast-food Mexican place is about as big as a blood sugar challenge can get. Portions are generally huge, the tortillas used for burritos are larger than your head and filled with a cup or more of white rice, and the entrées tend to be loaded with more cheese calories than you usually consume in two meals combined. Thread your way around these potholes, and you can arrive at a delicious, healthy meal.

Ask the server to take away the tortilla chips. The Mexican equivalent of a big breadbasket is either a bowl of chips or nacho chips covered with cheese. Just say no.

Order a healthy starter instead. Look for ceviches (marinated raw fish or seafood); guacamole, which is full of good fats (ask for soft tortillas instead of deep-fried chips to dip, and don't overeat them); gazpacho, a spicy cold vegetable soup; black bean soup; and tortilla soup (chicken in broth with vegetables and thin fried tortilla chips). Ask for extra salsa for the table and eat it with a spoon rather than on chips.

For an entrée, look to fajitas. These are made with lean beef (or chicken or shrimp) grilled with onions and peppers. Other good choices are grilled chicken or fish dishes.

Order tacos and burritos as a bowl. Ask the server to go light on the rice and heavy on the veggies.

Go for soft tacos and tortillas. Hard tacos are fried, so you're better off with soft tacos. Request corn or whole wheat tortillas, if available, for more fiber. A small tortilla is the equivalent of a slice of bread. If you're not eating rice, two or three soft tacos are fine, but stick to one or two if you are having rice. If you're getting a burrito, ask for no rice and more beans.

As a side dish, go for rice and beans instead of Mexican rice. Thanks to the beans, this dish has a lower glycemic load than rice alone. But check first to be sure the beans aren't refried. Refried beans are likely loaded with fat.

Have dessert at home. Desserts at Mexican restaurants, such as flan and fried ice cream, are usually high in calories and fat, so skip them and eat something healthier elsewhere.

WHAT TO ORDER

■ Appetizers/Sides
Tortilla soup; gazpacho; rice and beans (not refried); soft tortillas with salsa.

■ Entrées
Chicken or steak fajitas; soft chicken tacos (portion: two tacos); chicken or bean burrito; grilled chicken or fish; grilled chicken salad without the taco bowl.

WHAT NOT TO ORDER

■ Appetizers/Sides
Tortilla chips; nachos; quesadillas; refried beans.

■ Entrées
Taco salads; hard-shell tacos; chimichangas; beef or cheese enchiladas; beef burritos; chile rellenos; anything "grande."

continued >>>

Eating Out Chinese

The traditional Chinese diet is a healthy one, with lots of vegetables, stir-fries with small chunks of meat or fish, and soy foods. But that's not evident in the typical fare in a Chinese restaurant here, where the meal is likely to be heavy on greasy meats and swimming in sauces with lots and lots of calories. Even the vegetables are usually laden with a fatty sauce. Here's your game plan.

Ask for brown rice. Many restaurants give you the option. And don't eat the whole bowl or container of rice. Spoon a half cup onto your plate and leave the rest. Or do as a Chinese native would: Put a small amount in a small bowl and hold the bowl up, using your chopsticks (or fork) to eat a little rice in between bites of your main dish. Or be bold and don't eat any rice at all.

Start your meal with wonton or egg-drop soup. This will take the edge off your hunger without a lot of calories (avoid soups with coconut milk). If you want a ravioli-type appetizer, order steamed vegetable dumplings, but nothing fried.

When it comes to entrées, order from the "healthy" menu. Here is where you'll find steamed chicken and vegetables with sauce on the side and similar low-fat choices. Another good choice is moo goo gai pan (chicken with mushrooms). If you like stir-fries, ask the waitperson to have yours prepared with less oil and more veggies, and get the sauce on the side.

Make sure you order plenty of vegetables. If you really want to make the meal healthier, order a plate of steamed vegetables and add them to other dishes. Or ask for sautéed vegetables or Szechuan-style string beans.

Take advantage of the bean curd (tofu). Ordering family-style? Include a heart-healthy, low-fat dish such as bean curd with sautéed Chinese mixed vegetables (ask for sautéed bean curd, not deep-fried).

Plan to take home leftovers. Portions are often large. Think of about one cup of a dish (without rice) as a serving. Ask for a take-out container right away, so you can store the rest out of sight.

WHAT TO ORDER

■ Appetizers/Sides
Wonton soup; egg-drop soup; steamed dumplings; bok choy.

■ Entrées
Moo goo gai pan; chicken chow mein; steamed chicken with broccoli, sauce on the side; steamed chicken with mixed vegetables; bean curd (tofu) with mixed vegetables.

WHAT NOT TO ORDER

■ Appetizers/Sides
Hot-and-sour soup; velvet corn chowder; egg rolls; fried wonton; fried dumplings.

■ Entrées
General Tso's chicken; Kung Pao chicken; cashew chicken; moo shu pork; orange beef; spicy eggplant (eggplant soaks up oil).

Fast Food Without Fear

An occasional visit to a fast-food joint never killed anyone. Burgers and fries are still the staples on these menus, but the restaurants are now offering a greater selection of healthier fare. True, you'll have trouble locating a decent vegetable, other than salads, but you can keep the fat and calorie damage under control by ordering grilled sandwiches, salads, and even vegetarian burgers, chili, soup, and low-fat dairy desserts. Aim to make your meals "fast" ones less than once a week.

Opt for simple grilled fare, if you can find it. If there's a grilled chicken sandwich and the chicken isn't breaded, that's a good start. If you can, order it without mayonnaise or creamy sauces. This can save 100 calories or more.

A simple hamburger isn't bad either—if you order the smallest one. At 220 calories, Wendy's Jr. Hamburger is a low-cal burger. (By contrast, a Burger King Double Whopper with Cheese has 1,010 calories.)

Order à la carte. A "value" meal that includes fries and a big soft drink is often cheaper, but it's no nutritional bargain—the total calories can top 1,000! Unless you drink diet soda, skip the soft drink and ask for water—or orange juice, hot tea, coffee, or low-fat milk—instead. If it's a special treat, get the fries but buy the smallest size.

Take advantage of the salads. Just skip the cheese, bacon bits, and other add-ons. Ask for vinaigrette dressing. Try a salad as an entrée.

WHAT TO ORDER

■ Appetizers/Sides/Drinks
Garden salad; baked potato; fruit and yogurt parfait; water; low-fat milk; unsweetened ice tea.

■ Entrées
Grilled chicken sandwich; grilled chicken salad (skip the crispy noodles); junior hamburger; veggie burger; soft chicken taco; soft steak taco.

WHAT NOT TO ORDER

■ Appetizers/Sides/Drinks
French fries (if you must, order the small); hash browns; thick shakes; regular soda; sweetened iced tea.

■ Entrées
Double burgers; burgers with cheese or bacon; fried chicken sandwich; fried fish sandwich.

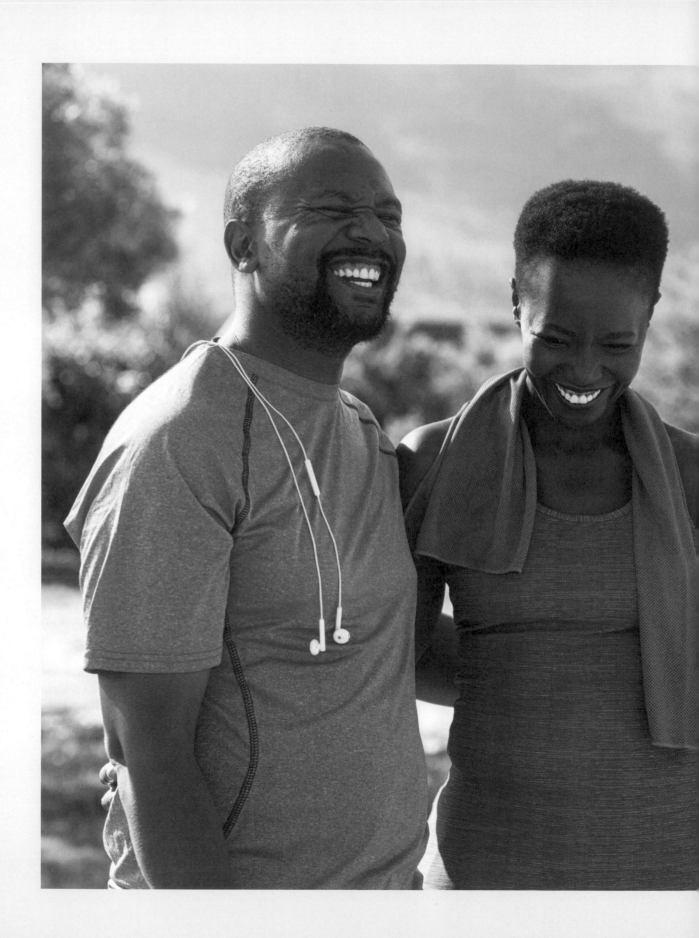

2

MOVE
to Reverse Diabetes

- Fitness Walking
- Easy Everyday Activity
- Simple Strength Moves

The Plan

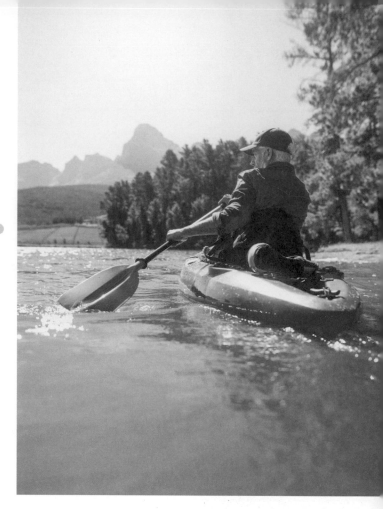

Easy and effective, our research-based Move to Reverse Diabetes plan stacks the deck in favor of better diabetes management. It does naturally what some drugs do: sensitizes cells to insulin so they soak up more glucose. Follow the plan for 12 weeks and you'll almost certainly see lower blood sugar levels. Your body will also burn more calories all day long, which means extra fat will come off more readily.

What to Do

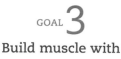

GOAL 1
Know how to exercise safely with diabetes

Exercise can make or break your efforts to lose weight and control your blood sugar—but when you have diabetes, you need to make sure you're exercising smartly and safely. It's important to guard against hypoglycemia (blood sugar that dips too low), to protect your feet, and, especially if you take insulin, to time your workouts.

GOAL 2
Walk at least five days a week

The core of the Move plan is a walk in the park, or around the neighborhood, or on a treadmill. Putting one foot in front of the other is a simple yet powerful way to meet *Reverse Diabetes'* twin goals of lower blood sugar and weight loss. Start with just 10 minutes a day and build up to 45-minute walks—energizing, calorie- and fat-burning workouts that feel great.

GOAL 3
Build muscle with the Sugar Buster Routine

Muscle mass is the secret to all-day blood sugar control and to maintaining a healthy weight with ease. Our Sugar Buster moves are safe, easy on your joints, and can be done in small pockets of downtime. You'll ease into the Sugar Buster Routine in Week 4 of our program and build up to performing all nine exercises twice each week.

GOAL 4
Make active choices every day

Equally important on the Move plan, you'll put everyday physical activity back into your life. Studies show that making active choices, from doing lawn work to going bowling, is a no-sweat way to lose weight and reduce your risk for diabetes and other health problems. We'll show you how to energize your life and burn hundreds of extra calories each day.

What to Record

1. THE NUMBER OF MINUTES YOU WALK EACH DAY

How much should you walk? "Your Goals Week by Week," below, outlines your exercise assignments. If you choose to wear a pedometer and count your steps every day, write your steps down, too. Record these on the habit trackers beginning on page 146.

2. WHETHER YOU PERFORMED THE SUGAR BUSTER EXERCISES

Beginning in Week 4 you'll add the Sugar Buster exercises to your weekly routine. Your ultimate goal is to perform the whole series of exercises twice each week. You can accomplish your goal in any way that fits your schedule.

3. OTHER EXERCISE YOU GET

Every time you make an active choice instead of an inactive choice during your day, give yourself a pat on the back by writing it down. That includes small stuff, such as taking the stairs instead of the elevator, and bigger stuff, such as mowing the lawn or playing a game of softball in the backyard. Recording these choices will motivate you to get up and move even more often.

Your Goals Week by Week

New to exercise? Short on time? No worries. The Move plan will ease you into a comfortable exercise routine that won't make you crazy.

WEEK	WALKING TIME	SUGAR BUSTER ROUTINE
1	10 minutes, five days a week	None
2	15 minutes, five days a week	None
3	20 minutes, five days a week	None
4	25 minutes, five days a week	Do each sequence once*
5	25 minutes, five days a week	Do each sequence once
6	30 minutes, five days a week	Do the entire routine twice
7	30 minutes, five days a week	Do the entire routine twice
8	35 minutes, five days a week	Do the entire routine twice
9	35 minutes, five days a week	Do the entire routine twice
10	40 minutes, five days a week	Do the entire routine twice
11	40 minutes, five days a week	Do the entire routine twice
12	45 minutes, five days a week	Do the entire routine twice

*choose a different day for each

Before You Begin

1 **Take the quiz on page 90**
It will help you assess your current fitness level, your attitude toward physical activity, and whether you're ready to find ways to fit more fitness into your day. Remember, these questions are for your eyes only. Answer as accurately as you can. You'll uncover valuable information that will help you customize the Move plan to fit your personality, your likes and dislikes, and your schedule.

2 **Read the safety information under Goal #1**
There you'll find a thorough discussion about exercising safely with diabetes. Read and digest the information before you start the plan.

3 **Buy a good pair of walking shoes**
High blood sugar and circulation problems mean that people with diabetes are at high risk for slow-healing sores that can lead to dangerous infections. That's why good walking shoes aren't a luxury for people with diabetes—they're a necessity. Turn to page 95 for advice.

The Quiz

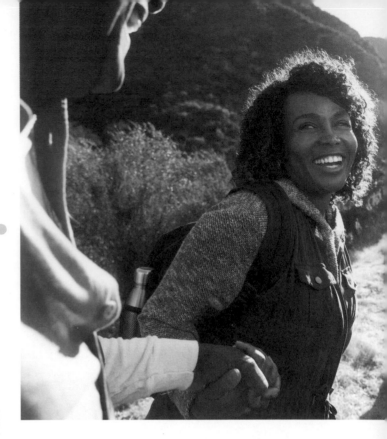

Are you ready to harness the power of movement to beat diabetes? This short quiz will help you understand where you stand—mentally, emotionally, and physically—when it comes to using physical activity to lower your blood sugar, lose weight, and beat stress.

Scan to take this quiz online.

1. My opinion about walking is:

a. It's a slow but cheap mode of transportation. Period.

b. It's probably good for you, but it's certainly not serious exercise.

c. It's a legitimate form of exercise I should do more.

d. It's not only great exercise but also a wonderful source of relaxation and pleasure.

2. If the weather's nice, I might walk for this long:

a. One minute—the time it takes to get from my car to the supermarket entrance.

b. Five minutes—the time it takes to find a nice bench in the park.

c. Twenty minutes—a relaxed stroll in the sun is a rare but pleasant treat.

d. Thirty minutes or more—I jump at every chance to be outside and moving.

3. My favorite parking spot at the mall is:

a. I don't know; I shop online.

b. Right up front; I'll circle until a primo spot opens.

c. Relatively near; I don't mind a little extra walking.

d. The farthest lot; this gives me a chance to get in one more brisk stroll.

4. If I walked briskly for 15 minutes, I would feel:

a. Surprised. I never walk unless it's to get from the house to the car or the car to the office or store.

b. As if someone knocked the wind out of me.

c. A little pooped, but still able to hold a conversation.

d. Invigorated and ready for another lap.

5. I would rate my strength as:

a. Low. When I get out of a chair, I have to push off using the armrests.

b. Not what it used to be; the grocery bags seem to weigh a ton, and I think twice before picking up small children.

c. Uneven. Some parts of my body are fairly strong, others are rather weak—even flabby.

d. Pretty darn good; I could lift a bag of potting soil or carry luggage.

6. When I think about exercise that builds muscle, I:

a. Don't think I need it. I'm not a bodybuilder.
b. Am intimidated by it—I worry that I'll have to go to a gym or lift heavy weights.
c. Am willing and interested but don't how to do it at home.
d. Have tried it and seen results—bring it on!

7. When I think about fitting exercise into my schedule, I:

a. Feel overwhelmed. I'm too busy already!
b. Guess I could trade a TV show for some exercise time but would rather not.
c. Know there are some things in my schedule that I could eliminate or streamline to make exercise a priority.
d. Have already cleared a dedicated exercise time most days of the week.

8. On a typical Saturday afternoon, I'm:

a. Watching the game on TV or otherwise deepening the depression in the seat of my chair.
b. Watching the kids' soccer or baseball game or driving around to do my errands.
c. Enjoying life—playing golf, bird-watching, doing something active with the kids or grandchildren.
d. Working in the yard, doing major housework or home repairs, or washing the car.

9. I've used exercise to lower my blood sugar in the following way:

a. I have to confess that I haven't tried it!
b. I've noticed that my blood sugar seems lower after I've been active, but I haven't made a conscious effort to use it that way.
c. I try to get regular exercise because it's good for my blood sugar, but I'm not consistent.
d. Not only do I exercise regularly to keep my blood sugar lower, I check my blood sugar before and after exercise to make sure it doesn't go too low.

10. My usual foot-care routine includes:

a. I don't pay any attention to my feet—who knows what's going on down there.
b. I glance at my feet after I bathe.
c. I try to wear the right shoes and to check my feet regularly.
d. I trim my toenails regularly, check my feet every day, and insist on wearing shoes that don't rub or pinch.

Your Score

Give yourself 1 point for each "a," 2 points for each "b," 3 points for every "c," and 4 points for each "d." Add your points together.

30–40 points
Hooray!
You're in gear. You're already living many aspects of the Move lifestyle. Now we'd like to challenge you to work your way up to 45 minutes of walking five days a week, and to set aside time for our muscle-strengthening Sugar Buster Routine twice a week. Doing these consistently will allow you to reap big rewards.

17–29 points
You're coasting.
You're interested in exercise, but tend to put other commitments—and others' expectations—first. Now's the time to renew your commitment to yourself and your health. Start by fitting in small bouts of exercise all day long (such as taking the stairs instead of the elevator) and setting aside time for fun physical activity, such as shooting some hoops or taking the grandkids to the park. Yes, these count as calorie-burning exercise—and they'll get you into the mindset for moving every day.

10–16 points
You're stalled.
Put the book down and take a 10-minute walk now. We want to prove to you that: a) You do have time for exercise; b) It doesn't take a major time commitment to reap the rewards of physical activity; and c) Exercise feels good—and fits into any schedule. Resolve to make time for yourself so that you can fit this important component of the Eat, Move, Choose plan into your life. Remind yourself of the benefits: better blood sugar control, a healthier weight, lower stress, and less risk for serious diabetes complications.

GOAL 1

Know how to exercise safely with diabetes

EXERCISE OFFERS such powerful blood sugar benefits it's almost like taking medicine. But just as you have to use medications judiciously and watch out for any side effects, you have to use exercise wisely and take steps to avoid problems such as low blood sugar and foot injuries. You'll also want to customize your workout plan to fit your personal needs and circumstances. Here's how.

STEP ONE
Talk with Your Team

Check with your doctor and registered dietitian or certified diabetes educator before starting any exercise program, especially if you're over age 35, have had diabetes for more than 10 years, or already show signs of heart disease, poor circulation, or nerve damage. Most people should have no problem with the exercises in this chapter. But it's worth a quick discussion. Here's what your conversation should cover.

Ask if you should take any special precautions. Ask if you have any diabetes-related conditions that would limit or change your routine.

For example, if an exercise stress test indicates heart trouble, you may be advised to walk at a more moderate pace. And if your feet have suffered nerve damage, you may be better off kicking in a pool than pounding the pavement.

Ask about side effects of any medications you take. Some oral diabetes medications can cause muscle ache or fatigue, while others can make you dizzy or nauseated. Be sure you and your doctor are clear about how intensely you intend to exercise and how your medication's side effects may limit your activities.

Ask if you need to change your diet. A registered dietitian or certified diabetes educator can help you determine the best way to fuel your personalized fitness routine.

STEP TWO
Learn How to Time Your Exercise

If you take insulin or oral diabetes drugs, it's important to time your exercise strategically so that blood sugar doesn't fall to dangerously low levels during your walk or workout. To ensure your safety, check with your doctor about taking steps such as the following.

Avoid peak hours for insulin and oral medications. Try to time your workout so that you're not exercising when the activity of insulin or pills peaks—often within the first hour or two of an injection or taking your diabetes medicines. This may be less of an issue for people who use insulin than it has been in the past. With the increased use of insulin pumps and intensive injection therapy, it's possible for people to exercise any time they can fit it in. Talk to your doctor or diabetes educator for specific advice.

If you're working to cut back on or eliminate your medication use, your doctor may start by having you take less (or none) before your workout. In effect, you may be able to exercise in place of taking your medication if the effects on your blood sugar prove to be similar.

Choose your injection site with care. If you inject insulin into muscles you'll be using, they will absorb it faster and send your blood sugar plummeting. Solution: Unless you're going straight into sit-ups, inject into the softer folds of your midsection. If you're working your abs, wait to exercise until about an hour after your injection to give the insulin a chance to disperse throughout the body.

Exercise after eating. Instead of relying on snacks to head off low blood sugar during your walk, be diligent about planning to exercise after a meal so that you can take advantage of higher, more sustained blood sugar levels.

STEP THREE

Test Your Blood Sugar Before, During, and After Exercise

Grab your blood-sugar meter and a test strip! Before you start to exercise, blood-sugar testing can

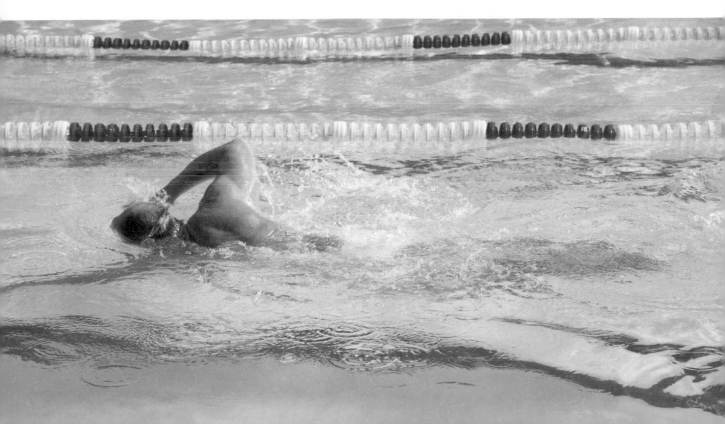

tell you when it might be better to hold off, at least until your glucose levels can meet your muscles' demands. It's wise to test your blood sugar again afterward, too, to see how far it's fallen. This will give you a sense of how exercise affects your blood sugar levels so that you can make adjustments in meals, snacks, and the timing of your exercise.

If you don't already keep a glucose log or track your levels on a diabetes management app, we've included a log on page 182 where you can record your daily food intake and physical activity to give you a clear picture of how your efforts

Scan to go to the log.

pay off. Make photocopies or, if you prefer, go to thehealthy.com/reversediabetes/foodexerciselog to find an digital copy you can fill out. Examine it and take note of any patterns.

Protect against hypoglycemia. Don't exercise

if your blood sugar is below 100 mg/dl. Instead, have a piece of fruit or other snack containing at least 15 grams of carbohydrate, then test again in about 20 minutes. Keep snacking until blood sugar rises above the 100 mg/dl mark.

Protect against hyperglycemia. Test for ketones using a urine ketone test strip if blood sugar before exercise is above 240 mg/dl. If the test detects ketones, don't start exercising until you've taken more insulin to handle glucose uptake during your workout. If ketones are absent, don't exercise if blood sugar is above 400 mg/dl.

Drink plenty of water. Get a water bottle that you like and that's easy to carry. Take it with you during your walks and sip regularly, especially when you're feeling thirsty.

STEP FOUR

Be Prepared for Low Blood Sugar Emergencies

Exercise works so well at bringing down your blood sugar that you need to make sure it doesn't drop *too* low. Hypoglycemia can happen even if you've planned carefully, so it's important to be prepared for this emergency. Here's how.

Know the signs of low blood sugar—and when to stop exercising. Confusion, shaking, lightheadedness, or difficulty speaking all indicate that you should quit exercising *immediately* and take steps to stabilize your glucose level. We can't stress this enough. When you first detect symptoms of hypoglycemia, don't wait "just one more minute" or "a while longer to see if symptoms improve." True, some symptoms can be confusing: Sweating and a rapid heartbeat could be a natural response to exercise—or signs of hypoglycemia. It's always wise to err on the side of safety.

The Blood Sugar Paradox

Why does blood sugar go down sometimes but go up other times after exercise? Muscles use glucose for energy, so as a rule, blood sugar goes down when you're active, as the body moves glucose from the liver and bloodstream into the cells. But that assumes there's enough insulin on hand to help with this transfer. If you take insulin and your dose is too low, glucose can build in the blood during exercise and cause hyperglycemia. That's why it's important to consult your doctor for advice on exercising and to check your blood sugar before and after (and perhaps even during) exercise to understand how physical activity affects you.

Carry the right snack with you. A small carbohydrate snack can bring blood sugar back up in an emergency—but only if you remember to bring one with you every time you walk. When blood sugar dips too low, bring it back up with 10 small jellybeans or the number of glucose tablets your doctor or certified diabetes educator suggests.

Check your blood sugar during long walks. When you're taking a long walk, stop and check your blood sugar after 30 minutes to make sure your blood sugar stays in your target range.

Use the buddy system. It's not always obvious when hypoglycemia is setting in (in fact, denying that anything's wrong can be a classic sign of early hypoglycemia), so it's wise to walk or work out with somebody else or in a place where other people are available if you need help, especially if you're exercising vigorously. Tell your workout partner what to watch for. If you work out at a gym, make sure the gym records indicate that you have diabetes.

Carry identification. Even if you're just strolling through the neighborhood, carry ID with your name, address, phone number, contact information for your doctor and a family member, and the names and dosages of your medication or insulin.

Stay alert afterward. Blood sugar can continue to fall long after you've exercised, so don't let your guard down for signs of hypoglycemia until 24 hours after your workout.

STEP FIVE
Have a Foot-Protection Plan

The feet can take a beating when you have diabetes. Poor circulation from damaged blood vessels slows healing and makes feet more prone to infection, while nerve damage can dull sensation and

Foot hassles may seem mundane, but you can't dismiss them if you have diabetes.

leave you oblivious to injuries that can quickly get out of control. Foot hassles may seem mundane, but you just can't dismiss broken skin, corns, calluses, bunions, or ingrown toenails when you have diabetes. Left untreated for long, such conditions can put you at risk of losing a foot—or even a leg—to gangrene. In fact, about 15 percent of people with diabetes in the United States eventually develop foot problems that threaten a limb, and more than 50,000 must undergo amputations every year. Don't be one of those people.

Buy the right pair of walking shoes. The sole piece of equipment you need on the Move plan is a good pair of walking shoes. They'll help you travel farther and faster with more comfort—and no blisters or injuries.

Shop at a respected athletic-shoe store. A skilled salesperson can size your feet and find the best shoe for your foot shape and size. Tell the

That's Easy!

At medical appointments, take off your socks and shoes even if your doctor doesn't tell you to. Your feet should be examined at every visit for signs of skin breakdown, hot spots, cracked heels, or ingrown toenails. If you keep a glucose log book, put it between your toes. This way you'll be sure that both your feet and your log book will be examined!

salesperson what type of terrain you'll be walking on and how many miles you plan to walk. If you usually shop online, consider visiting a brick-and-mortar shoe store at least once to get sized and fitted. After determining the best shoe for you, you can then purchase replacement pairs online.

Bring an old pair of walking shoes to the store. The salesperson can look at the wear pattern on your shoes to determine what type of shoe you need. For example, if the inner heel is more worn than the outer heel, you'll want extra arch support and a shoe designed for "motion control."

Try on your shoes and walk around the store. Wear the socks you plan to walk in. Make sure the shoe hugs your heel; your heel should not slide up and down as you walk. The shoe should also have a firm arch support, and the forefoot of the shoe should bend with the natural bend in your foot. Most important, the shoes should feel comfortable when you walk.

Do the twist test. A good walking shoe should be flexible enough to accommodate your foot's natural heel-to-toe roll. If you can't twist the sole from side to side, it's too stiff.

Examine your feet daily. If you have nerve damage, you could have sores, cuts, swelling, and infection that you can't feel, so give your feet an exam once a day, perhaps at bedtime. Go over them with both your eyes and your hands. Let your doctor know if you find evidence of any problems. Besides blisters, cuts, bruises, cracking, or peeling, look for areas that are shaded differently (either paler or redder), which could indicate persistent pressure from shoes. Feel for areas of coldness, which could be a sign of poor circulation, or warmth (along with redness), which might be evidence of an infection. If you have trouble seeing the bottoms of your feet, place a mirror on the floor and look at the reflection.

Clean and treat minor scrapes and cuts right away. If you find a small cut or sore on your foot, treat it immediately. Wash your hands with soap and water. Then wash the wound with soap and water, rinse with more water, and pat it dry with a clean towel or tissue paper. Dab some antibiotic ointment onto a cotton swab and smear a thin layer of the ointment onto the wound. (Don't apply the ointment with your finger.) Cover the wound with an adhesive bandage. If the wound doesn't look better within a day, or if you see signs of infection, such as swelling, redness, warmth, or oozing, call your doctor or podiatrist immediately.

Keep your tootsies smooth and dry. Avoid cracked skin and reduce the risk of infection by toweling off your feet thoroughly after bathing, especially between your toes. Rub lotion or cream on the tops and bottoms of your feet to keep them moist, and sprinkle talcum or talc-free powder between your toes to prevent fungal growth.

Trim your toenails. Do it at least once a week after bathing, cutting straight across the nails and smoothing them with a nail file or emery board. If this is difficult for you, ask your podiatrist to trim your toenails or treat yourself to a pedicure.

GOAL 2

Walk at least five days a week

IT'S TIME TO HIT YOUR STRIDE! Starting today, lace up a good pair of sneakers or walking shoes and head out the door. Why walking? It's something almost anyone can do, almost anywhere. It costs nothing. It's a great excuse to get outside, something most of us do too infrequently. (Remember that practically any weather is good walking weather as long as you're dressed for it.)

On the Move plan you'll build to 45 minutes of walking five times a week. But for now, the important thing is to get out there—and build a routine you'll love so much you can't live without it. Start as slowly as you like. Gradually you'll pick up the pace and add to the length of your walks, so that by Week 10 you'll be working your heart and muscles enough to really make a difference. Here's how to fit walking in

STEP ONE
Find the Perfect Time and Place

Customizing your walking routine so that it fits your schedule and your preferences can make the difference between success and *oops... I didn't fit my walk in again today.* There's no one-size-fits-all solution, no time of day or location that works for everyone—and that's the true beauty of walking. Whatever works for you is the right way to do it, whether you decide to start by fitting in a couple of 10-minute strolls in-between job, home, and other activities; walking on a treadmill during your favorite TV show; or indulging in a long, brisk jaunt in a scenic park. Walking is the centerpiece of the Move plan, and if you make it work for you, you'll be able to stick with it come what may. Here are some strategies for making it happen.

Roll out of bed, get dressed, put on your shoes, and go. It's easy to get caught up in your day-to-day activities and tell yourself that you don't have time for a walk. If you exercise first thing in the morning, however, you will have no need for excuses. Research shows that people who plan to exercise in the morning are more likely to fit in their workouts than people who plan to exercise later in the day. And exercising in the morning may offer a side benefit: You'll sleep better at night. When researchers at the Fred Hutchinson

Cancer Research Center in Seattle, Washington, compared morning and evening exercise, people who exercised at least 225 minutes per week in the morning had an easier time falling asleep at night than those who completed the same amount of exercise in the evening.

Or, walk in the evening. That sleep study aside, we still like after-dinner walks. They get you away from the television and keep you from eating too much at dinner, and it's just a lovely time of day. Don't let unlovely weather stop you either—that's what jackets, boots, and umbrellas were invented for. There's something childlike and fun about a walk in the rain or snow.

Split it up. When you're too busy to go for your usual 30- or 45-minute walk, divide and conquer.

Get out there for five or 10 minutes at a time. That may be as simple as taking a five-minute walk break around the building after completing a project at work. Such short walking breaks will refresh your mind so you can return to work with more vigor. In fact, research shows that most of us can focus at top capacity for only 30 minutes at a time. After that, concentration begins to drop off. Your intermittent walk breaks may make you more productive.

Try a treadmill. If the mail carrier can deliver mail in any weather, you can walk in any weather, as long as you're dressed for it. But if you live in a climate that's often too hot or too cold for comfort, consider joining a gym or investing in a treadmill.

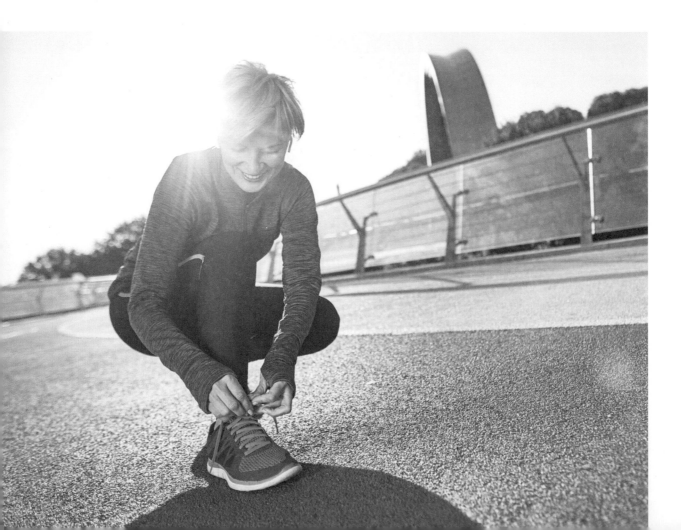

STEP TWO

Set Your Pace

If you already walk for exercise, picking up the pace can help you get fit faster, according to a slew of scientific studies. In an eight-year analysis of 72,488 female nurses ranging in age from 40 to 65, researchers found that those who worked up a sweat for just 90 minutes a week—the equivalent of about 12 minutes a day—lowered their risk for chronic health conditions such as diabetes and heart disease by 30 to 40 percent. Similarly, a Harvard Health Professionals study of 44,452 men ages 40 to 79 found that those who ran for an hour or more each week dropped their heart disease risk by 42 percent.

You don't have to (and should not) heave and gasp and hurt to reap these rewards. New exercisers can raise their heart rates into the vigorous zone with little more than brisk walking. When University of Massachusetts researchers asked 84 overweight people to walk one mile at a pace that was "brisk but comfortable," the vast majority of the volunteers stepped right up to an average 3.2-mph pace, which translates into hard to very hard intensity (70 to 100 percent of their maximum heart rates). The best part? It was easier than people expected, the researchers report.

Here's how to set the right pace, whether you're a beginning fitness walker or a veteran.

Beginners: Take it slow and easy. Your top priority is regular walking, not setting new speed records. Be sure that you're comfortable with your routine and that it fits into your life, even on busy days. If you're new to walking or haven't hit the pavement for a while, or if your doctor—or your body—tells you to start slowly, we recommend beginning with baby steps. Walk for just 10 minutes at a comfortable pace and gradually, over the next few weeks, build up to 20 minutes. Then pick up the pace.

Three Ways to
Get Yourself Walking

We get it—new habits take time to form. Use these strategies to get in the habit of walking five days a week.

- **Walk while doing something else you love.** Like podcasts or audio books? Fire one up while you walk. Known as "temptation bundling," pairing an activity you want to do (listening to that podcast or book) with a behavior you're struggling to do (walking) can help you walk 51 percent more frequently, according to research done by Katy Milkman, a professor of behavior change at the University of Pennsylvania.

- **Use your lunch break.** Eat lunch at your desk, then take a walk around the building or the block. You'll have more energy for the afternoon—and will be more likely to avoid hitting the vending machine for a pick-me-up. Bonus: Research finds that just six minutes of walking is enough to perk up your mood, helping you to tackle the afternoon with gusto.

- **Be your own cheerleader.** Too often, we focus on the negative, telling ourselves things such as "I only walked for five minutes" and "Gosh my pace was slow." That negative self talk can be discouraging, making us less likely to want to walk in the future. Instead, look for wins, no matter how small, and celebrate them. Did you put your walk in your calendar for the first time ever? Yay you! No win is too small to celebrate.

Always warm up first. Start every walk with five minutes of easy-paced walking—about the same pace at which you'd do your grocery shopping—to get your body warmed up. Then, cool down at the end of each walk with another five minutes of easy-paced walking. This allows your heart rate to gradually speed up and slow down.

Breathe deeply as you walk to a count of 1-2-3. Many people unintentionally hold their breath when they exercise and then suddenly feel breathless and tired. Oxygen is invigorating, and muscles need oxygen to create the energy for movement. So as you inhale, bring the air to the deepest part of your lungs by expanding your tummy and inhale for a count of three. Then exhale fully either through your nose or mouth, also to the count of three.

Take the talk test. Once you're walking 20 minutes or more each day, aim for a brisk pace—the speed you'd reach if you were 10 minutes late for an appointment. If you're able to recite the Pledge of Allegiance without hesitating, your exercise level is easy. If you can get it out phrase by phrase with little pauses for breath in between, you're right on target. If you can barely make it to "to the flag" without gasping for air, you're working too hard (that said, if you're in good shape and your heart is healthy, it's OK to exercise in this heart-rate zone, but only for a few minutes at a time).

Walking for 30 minutes or longer? Add in faster bursts. Incorporating brief bursts of faster walking during your walks helps you burn more fat and calories in the same amount of time. Move at your usual speed for three to five minutes, then walk even more briskly for one to two minutes. To pick up the pace, take short, quick steps. (Most people try to walk faster by elongating their strides, but this actually slows you down and can lead to joint and shin injuries.) Bend your arms at 90 degrees and pump them quickly. After your fast-walking interval, settle back into your usual brisk pace for three to four minutes, then pick up the pace again for one to two minutes. Do this several times during your walk. Boosting the intensity intermittently—known as high-intensity interval training, or HIIT—can increase your calorie burn by as much as 60 percent.

That's Easy!

Don't feel like walking? Vow to walk for just 10 minutes, and head out the door. Chances are, once you've warmed up, you'll exercise for longer than you anticipated. Even if you don't, 10 minutes is better than no minutes at all. You'll lower your blood sugar, burn calories, and maintain this important fitness habit.

STEP THREE
Stay Motivated

Once you're up and moving, maintain your momentum. Some people revel in the ritual of walking the same route at the same time every day. But for most of us, variety is the key to staying interested. These steps will keep your foot-powered plan fun and inspiring.

Walk with a friend. If she's expecting you, you're more likely to get out of bed on cold winter mornings or skip the cafeteria in favor of a lunchtime walk. If one of you backs out for any reason, put $5 in a kitty. Hopefully this will never happen, but if you build up a substantial sum, donate it to charity.

Pick a charity. Sign up for a charity walk or choose a cause or nonprofit you believe in—such as breast cancer research, the American Red Cross, the United Way—and for the next two weeks, pledge to contribute $1 for every mile you walk. You'll take pride in the fact that you are walking for something beyond yourself, which will motivate you to go longer and faster. After every walk, make a note on your phone of the amount you own (or post it on social media). When you reach $50, make a donation online. Whoever thought exercise could be tax deductible?

Walk for entertainment one day a week. Instead of walking around your neighborhood,

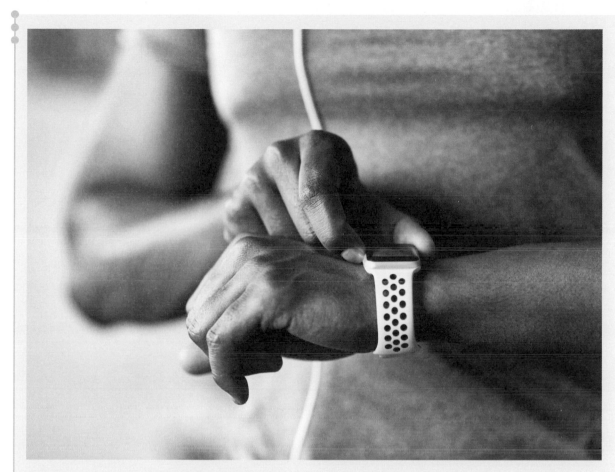

Make Every Step Count

To motivate yourself to walk more, consider using the step counter that most likely came for free with your smart phone or smart watch. Alternatively, you can purchase an inexpensive pedometer that clips to your waistband. Here's how to use it.

Establish your baseline. On a typical day before beginning the Move program, make sure to have your step counter with you everywhere you go. At the day's end, note how many steps you took. That's your baseline. You'll quickly discover that everyday activities such as taking out the trash use about 100 steps per minute. So does strolling at a lively pace while shopping at the supermarket or mall. Hustling to an appointment tallies about 130 steps per minute.

Start walking. We recommend that you follow the walking plan even if you're also counting steps. It automatically increases your walking time over the 12-week program—and automatically boosts your step count. We estimate that the plan's fitness walk will add about 1,250 steps for every 10 minutes of walking you do.

Go for "extra credit" steps. If your daily activities plus a walk don't add up to 5,000 steps, find opportunities to step out throughout the day. Park farther from the supermarket entrance, walk the mall before you begin shopping, or play a little longer with the dog, the kids, or the grandchildren. Every step counts.

Your top priority is regular walking, not setting speed records.

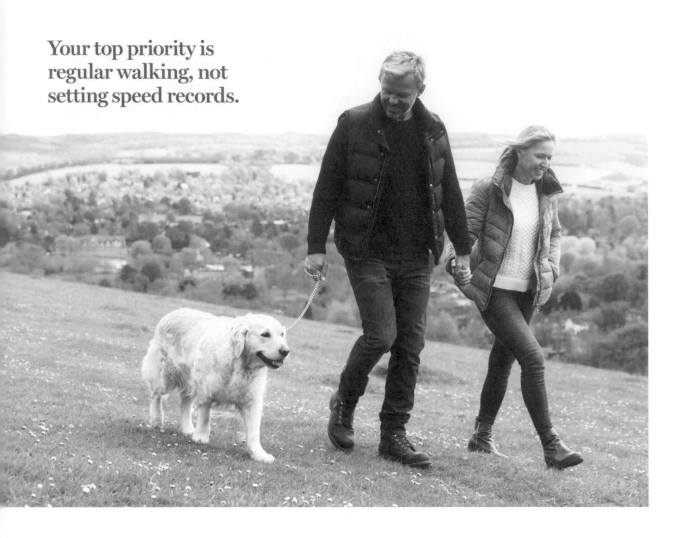

walk through the zoo, an art museum, or an upscale shopping mall. First circle the perimeter of your location at your usual brisk pace. Then wander through again more slowly to take in the sights.

Take the entire family on your daily walks. Not only will you be modeling good fitness habits for your children, but you'll also be able to supervise them while you walk rather than getting a sitter. If your children walk too slowly, ask them

to ride their bikes or roller-skate alongside you. To keep everyone entertained, play your usual repertoire of long car trip games, such as "I Spy." You can also try a scavenger walk, where you start out with a list of items to find during your walk and check off the list as you spot them.

Once a week, complete your errands on foot. If you live within a mile of town, or even a convenience store, start from your house. If you live out in the middle of nowhere, drive to within a mile

Sugar Buster Quiz

Q: Sidewalks or dirt paths?

A: Dirt paths.

If you're over 60, walk on soft surfaces. As you age, the fat padding in your feet deteriorates. The absence of this natural shock absorber can make walking on sidewalks and other hard surfaces feel like foot torture. Flat grass and dirt paths will provide more cushioning for your feet than roads or sidewalks.

Posture Perfect

Improving your walking posture will help you burn more fat and calories and help prevent muscle and joint pain. Readjust yourself to the following standards:

▶ Stand tall with your spine elongated and your breastbone lifted. This allows room for your lungs to fully expand.

▶ Keep your head straight with your eyes focused forward and your shoulders relaxed. Avoid slumping your shoulders forward or hunching them toward your ears.

▶ Roll your feet from heel to toe.

▶ As you speed up, take smaller, more frequent steps. This protects your knees and gives your butt a good workout.

▶ Allow your arms to swing freely.

▶ Firm your tummy and flatten your back as you walk to prevent low back pain.

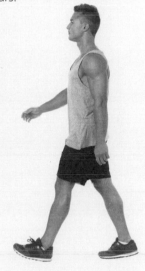

of your destination, park, and walk the rest of the way there and back. You'll be surprised how much you can accomplish on foot, and even better, how many people you'll meet along the way.

Explore your world. Spy on the new houses going up in the development nearby. Try walking down a street in your own neighborhood that you've never been on (and say hi to the neighbors you've never met). Or check out the hiking trail in a nearby park. Varying your terrain will do more than keep you mentally engaged. It will also help you to target different leg muscles, improving the effectiveness of every outing.

Take a dog with you. Once your dog gets used to your walks, he or she will look forward to them and give you a gentle nudge (or annoying whine) on the days you try to get out of it. There's nothing more effective than a set of puppy dog eyes to extract your butt from the couch and get it out the door. Don't have a dog? Offer to walk an elderly neighbor's dog twice a week. That commitment will keep you motivated.

Pump up the volume. Research proves it: Listening to music while walking helps you walk longer, probably because you're distracted by the

songs and almost forget that you're exercising. So load up your favorite tunes, especially those with a fast beat, and plug yourself in! Just be sure to keep the volume low enough that you can hear traffic and stay aware of your surroundings.

Join an online fitness community. Many fitness apps not only help you count steps and provide you with workout tips, but also give you access to an online fitness community that can help cheer you on and keep you moving.

GOAL 3

Build muscle with the Sugar Buster Routine

IMAGINE KEEPING your blood sugar in better control all day long, even when you're sleeping, taking in the latest James Bond movie, or sipping a cup of coffee with a friend. You can accomplish this feat if you invest just a little bit of time in building up your muscles. Using your muscles forces your muscle cells to soak up more glucose. The bonus: You'll look trimmer, have more energy for daily tasks such as carrying groceries or grandkids, and even improve your balance.

Building sexy, sugar-sipping muscles is the goal you'll achieve if you follow the plan's Sugar Buster Routine. This set of nine exercises couldn't be simpler. All you need is a pair of sneakers, comfortable clothing, and a few everyday objects: a towel or exercise mat for exercises done while sitting or lying on the floor; a chair, table, or countertop for support for a few moves; and the stairs in your home.

Once you've mastered the moves and they become easy, you can add light hand weights or ankle weights if you'd like, but right now working against your own body weight is all you need. That also means you can do these exercises anywhere— in a hotel room while you're traveling, behind your office door at work, or in your living room, bedroom, or TV room.

Turn back to Your Goals Week by Week on page 89 to remind yourself how and when to ease into the routine (start in Week 4 of the Eat, Move, Choose Plan). When you perform any part of the routine, remember to record it—give yourself credit where credit is due!

Getting Started

The investment you need to make in order to reap the blood sugar and weight loss benefits of strength training may be smaller than you think. The routine that we've designed can be done in about 20 minutes—roughly the time you'd spend watching commercials during a typical hour-long TV show—so it's easy to do this workout during your favorite program.

The timing. We've broken the workout into three sequences, which take about five to seven minutes each, so that in the beginning weeks, you can do just one sequence on a particular day. You might do the Upper Body sequence on Monday, the Core

Body sequence on Wednesday, and the Lower Body sequence on Saturday, for instance. The three moves in each sequence don't even have to be done at the same time. You could spend just a couple of minutes doing one move in the morning, then spend a few more minutes doing the other two moves in the evening. As you get stronger, start doing the whole routine at once, and do it twice a week.

The rules. Both efficient and effective, the Sugar Buster Routine includes basic exercises that will come easily regardless of your past experience or level of strength now. Perform 8 to 12 repetitions of each exercise, then rest for 30 to 60 seconds in between exercises. Once the moves become easy, you can add a second set of repetitions. You'll also find tips for taking many of these moves up a notch once you get strong enough that even two sets of repetitions are easy.

One suggestion: Don't repeat the same exercise two days in a row. Muscles need time to rest and repair themselves between strength-training sessions. You'll get better results if you give each muscle group a day or two off before working it again.

Building sexy, sugar-sipping muscles couldn't be simpler. You'll look trimmer, feel more energetic, and improve your balance!

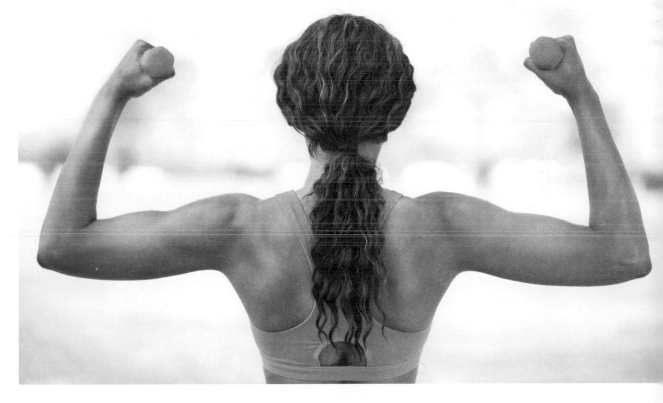

Upper Body Sequence

Wall Push-Up

This is easier than a regular push-up but does the same job.

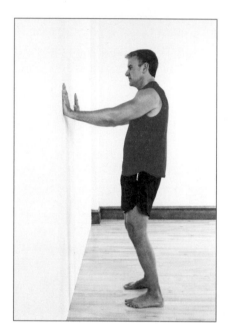

● **ONE** From a standing position about 12 to 18 inches from a wall, put your hands on the wall about shoulder-width apart at chest level, with palms flat and fingers pointed toward the ceiling.

● **TWO** Slowly lower your chin toward the wall. Smoothly push back from the wall to the starting position.

Smart Tip

As you lower yourself to the wall, keep your elbows out to the side. That works the chest muscles better than keeping elbows close to the body, which shifts the load more to the triceps muscles of the arms. If you feel pain in your hands or wrists, try placing your hands farther apart or closer together on the wall.

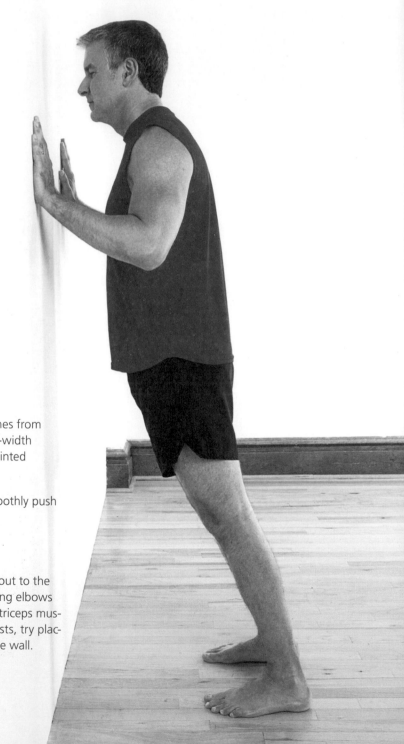

Armchair Dip

This is an exercise that encourages you to work muscles exactly the way you use them for everyday activities.

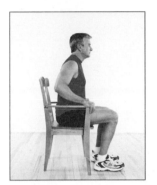 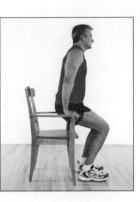

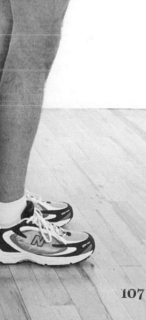

- **ONE** Sit in a sturdy armchair, back straight and feet flat on the floor about hip-width apart. Place your hands on the chair's arms about even with the front of your body.

- **TWO** Using mostly your arms but assisting with your legs, push yourself out of the chair to a full standing position, letting go of the chair as you stand.

- **THREE** Lower yourself back into the chair, putting your hands on the arms of the chair as you slowly come down, using your arm muscles to return to the starting position.

Smart Tip

For a variation, maintain your hold on the arms of the chair until you fully extend your arms, then slowly lower yourself back into the chair.

Seated Biceps Curl

This exercise for the biceps muscles will make hefting suitcases and heavy grocery bags a breeze and build shapely upper arms you won't mind baring in a sleeveless or short-sleeved shirt.

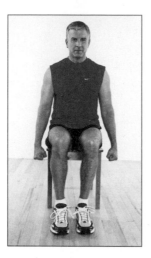

ONE Sit up straight on the front half of an armless chair, feet flat on the floor, with your arms hanging down by your side.

TWO Smoothly bend your elbows, keeping them positioned at your side, raising your hands toward your shoulders while rotating your palms a quarter turn so they face your shoulder at the top of the movement. Smoothly return to the starting position.

Smart Tip

If this exercise becomes too easy, try performing it while holding light dumbbells. Start with 1- or 2-pound weights.

Core Body Sequence

Bird Dog

This move works muscles of the hips, but also the back, chest, shoulders, and arms. The multi-element motion improves balance and coordination and helps promote good posture.

ONE Get down on your hands and knees on the floor, a rug, or an exercise mat.

TWO Extend your right leg out behind you, keeping your foot a few inches off the floor as you straighten your knee.

THREE At the same time as you extend your right leg, reach out straight in front of you with your left arm. Return to the starting position and repeat with the other leg and arm to complete one repetition.

FOUR Continue alternating legs and arms until you finish a set.

Smart Tip

Try to keep your back as flat as possible during the movement. If this exercise becomes too easy, try this variation: When you extend your leg behind you, raise it until it's parallel to the floor.

109

Abdominal Curl

The sit-up is a fundamental part of any well-rounded routine; this version is a little bit easier and also safer, but still effective for strengthening your abdominal muscles.

ONE Lie on your back with feet flat on the floor, knees bent, and arms folded across your chest, each hand touching the opposite shoulder.

TWO Raising your head, use your abdominal muscles to pull your shoulders off the floor so you can look at the top of your knees. Keep enough space to fit a baseball between your chin and chest.

THREE Slowly lower your shoulders back to the floor.

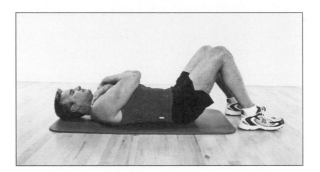

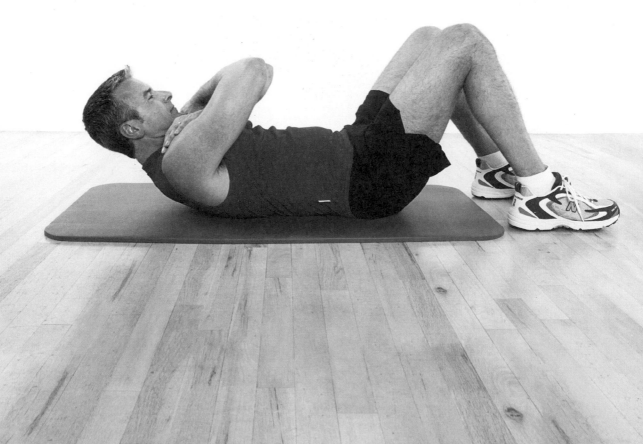

The Bicycle

This exercise is a favorite strength and endurance builder for athletes from football players to figure skaters. It helps tone the muscles along the sides of your abdomen, called the obliques.

ONE Lie flat on your back with your legs straight and your hands behind or lightly touching your ears.

TWO Lift your head off the floor and bring your left knee toward your head, stopping when your knee is about waist level and your thigh is perpendicular to the floor. At the same time, bring your right elbow toward the elevated knee so that your torso twists slightly and your elbow and knee are as close as possible over your abdomen.

THREE Slowly return to the starting position. Rest for one second and repeat with the opposite limbs.

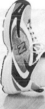

Smart Tip

This exercise should take about five seconds, with two seconds to bring knee and elbow close, and three seconds to return. As you become stronger, reduce the resting time for a more difficult workout. All motions should be smooth and controlled, which keeps longer resistance on muscles and improves strength and tone more quickly.

Lower Body Sequence

Stair Step-Up

This move helps build strong leg muscles and requires absolutely no equipment. Yes, you can use a special exercise step, but it's not necessary. A regular step in your home is preferable because you can lightly grasp the stair rail for support. To keep track of repetitions, count step-ups on just one foot.

- **ONE** Stand in front of a step with both feet on the floor about hip-width apart.

- **TWO** Place your right foot solidly on the stair and step up. Bring your left foot up and touch it lightly on the step before lowering it back to the floor.

- **THREE** Step down with your right foot.

- **FOUR** Step up with your left foot, bringing your right foot up and touching it lightly on the step, then lowering it back to the floor. Alternate steps in this way, counting one repetition when each foot has stepped up one time.

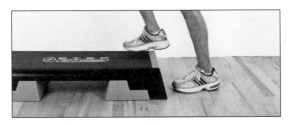

Smart Tip

Make this exercise more difficult by using only one foot instead of alternating. For example, use the right foot to step up, step down, then step up again rather than alternating with the left foot. When you've finished a set of step-ups with the right foot, do a set with the left.

Side Hip Abduction

This exercise works the abductor muscles on the outside of the hip and the outer thigh.

● **ONE** Lie on your right side with both legs extended and resting one on top of the other, supporting your head with your right hand.

● **TWO** In a smooth and controlled motion, lift your fully extended left leg straight up as high as you comfortably can. Then lower it back to the starting position. After one set, repeat with the other leg.

Smart Tip

If you feel unstable in the starting position, try bending the lower leg to provide a wider base of support. If this exercise becomes too easy, try performing it while wearing light ankle weights. Start with ½-pound or 1-pound weights.

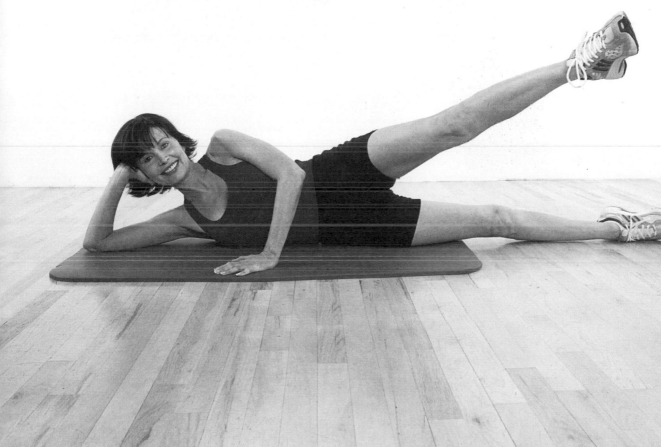

Standing Hip Extension

Perform this exercise facing a sturdy chair, countertop, or table you can rest your hands on for balance and support. It works your hips, buttocks, hamstrings, and lower back.

ONE Stand with feet about hip-width apart, lightly holding a chair or counter.

TWO Without bending the knee, move your right leg back behind you from the hip. Return slowly to the starting position. After one set, repeat with the other leg.

Smart Tip

Don't lock the knee of the leg you stand on, but instead keep it slightly bent. While the motion is pendulum-like, you shouldn't let momentum do the work. Perform the move slowly, especially during the return phase. If this exercise becomes too easy, try it with a light ankle weight.

GOAL 4

Make active choices every day

WHAT KIND OF EXERCISE can you do while stuck in a line at the grocery store, when you have to relay information to a coworker, or when it's time to entertain the kids or grandkids? How about small, stealthy, calorie-burning moves that also use up blood sugar and help you lose weight—without taking time out of your day?

Thanks to modern technology we've engineered so many old-fashioned "inconveniences" out of our lives that we're packing on pounds. That's why we've made living an active life an essential part of the Move plan. It's just as important as walking and strength training for helping you achieve and maintain a healthy weight and for keeping your blood sugar in check.

Rediscovering the joys of an active lifestyle is fun. We bet you'll find yourself figuring out loads of new ways to fit more activity into your day, whether you play kickball with the kids in the backyard; stand and pace rather than lounging on the couch during phone calls; bound up the stairs rather than taking the elevator; or volunteer to take the dog out for an extra walk.

This vivacious approach to daily life is also energizing—not energy-sapping, as the typical sedentary lifestyle typically is. When you make active choices, your appetite for movement and activity is whetted, making the rest of the Move plan easier and more enjoyable to follow. Here's how to start living the active life today.

STEP ONE

Seize Opportunities to Move Every Day

At home, at work, and everywhere in between, there are dozens of opportunities to move your body instead of sitting still. We've outlined just a few ideas; feel free to come up with more of your own.

At Work

Take energy breaks. Every half hour, walk around your office or down the hall for five minutes. Jump up and down in your own office. Do push-ups with your hands resting against your desk. Do 10 leg lifts, then stand up and rise on your toes 10 times. Stretch your arms high 10 times, too.

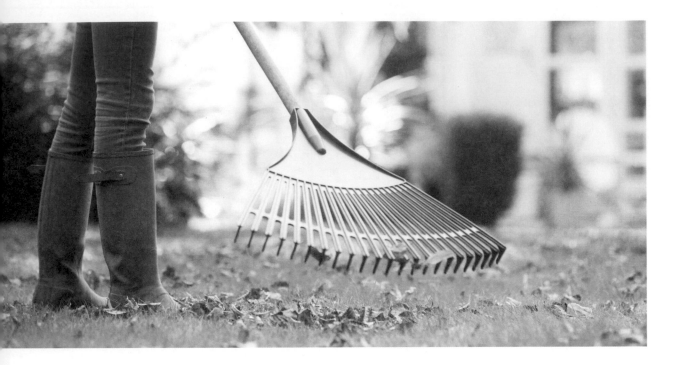

Get a new rolling "chair." Try sitting on a large exercise ball instead of a desk chair, at least some of the time. You'll use your abdominal and back muscles all day to help you balance.

Take the stairs. Just two flights daily could help you melt six pounds in a year. In fact, climbing stairs for two minutes five days a week provides the same calorie burn as a 36-minute walk.

Go the long way. Circle the building before heading to lunch. Use the bathroom farthest from your desk. Doesn't it feel good to stretch your legs?

Get more "face time." Instead of sending e-mails, stop by your coworkers' desks to ask a question. Doing this instead of sending just one e-mail a day could save you 11 pounds over 10 years. If you're working remotely, try a standing desk.

Plan a walking meeting. Need to schedule a small meeting? Suggest a walking meeting instead of a confab in an airless conference room. Chances are, you'll have better ideas and forge a better relationship with your fellow walkers—plus you can more easily practice social distancing if you need to.

At Home

Cook as if it's 1904. Chop veggies by hand instead of in the food processor, whip eggs with a fork or whisk, mix cake batter with a big spoon instead of the mixer, dig out your manual can opener, and, if you have time, wash and dry the dishes by hand. It will all add up to a small workout.

Rake leaves instead of using a leaf blower. You'll burn 50 more calories every half hour.

Scrub your floors more often. Putting some elbow grease into cleaning floors is more intense exercise than vacuuming—and it makes your floors look better to boot.

Spiff up your ride. Wash your car by hand. You'll save money by not going to the car wash and burn up to 280 calories in an hour. Why not vacuum the upholstery and carpeting and wash the plastic trim on the insides of the doors, too?

Trim the old-time way. Leave the electric edger and trimmer in the garage and grab your old hand tools. Comfort hint: Use thick foam or an old carpet square to cushion your knees.

Rehab the push mower. Revive a lovely summer sound: the *whisk-whisk-whisk* of a muscle-powered push mower. Sharpen the blades, oil the mechanism, and go. Ah! No exhaust fumes, no ugly power-motor noise.

Double-dig. Gardeners know that the best planting beds are double-dug. When you put in a new bed or turn over the soil in your vegetable patch in the spring, leave the power tiller in the shed and get out there with a sharp shovel. Dig each row twice—first to a single shovel's depth, then down one more shovel's worth. Refill the row by putting the first digging's soil in the bottom and the second's on top. You'll have more fertile soil on top and fluffy dirt down deep, so tender roots can grow strong, creating beautiful, healthy plants.

Plant bulbs. Garden catalogs start advertising sales of fall bulbs in midsummer. That's the time to think about daffodils, daylilies, tulips, and a host of other gorgeous spring and summer flowers for next year. Order a bunch and plant them over several fall weekends. Your efforts will be rewarded with a stunning display once winter's gone.

Stop buying weed killer. Be a friend to the earth and to your own muscles: Pull, dig out, and cut back weeds yourself. Your arms and back will get a workout.

Anytime, Anywhere

Hop on the escalator at the mall or train station, but walk instead of just taking a ride. You'll get there faster and use your muscles while you're at it. Just five minutes of stair climbing burns 144 calories.

Don't sit when you can stand. When cooling your heels while waiting in a doctor's office, drugstore, or airport, stay on your feet. Standing burns 36 more calories per hour than sitting.

STEP TWO

Sneak in "Stealth" Exercise Moves

Most of us hate to kill time, but we face countless opportunities during the day to do just that.

On the Road to Fitness: Car Moves

Reserve these fast, effective exercises for stoplights and long traffic jams.

Steering wheel lift press. While stopped at a red light, grasp the bottom of the steering wheel with your palms up. Inhale and then, while exhaling, push up on the wheel with your palms as hard as you can. Hold while breathing normally until the light turns green. This works the biceps, the primary load-bearing muscles of the arms.

Ab squeeze. While stopped at a red light or stop sign, take a deep breath through your mouth, dropping your diaphragm so your stomach pushes out. While exhaling, squeeze your abdominal muscles so your back presses into the car seat. (Imagine that a hook around your spine is pulling you back.) Hold for up to 60 seconds while breathing normally. This improves posture and tones abs to support your back and make you look slimmer.

Opportunities? That's right: From now on, be alert for small moments of downtime during your day and embrace them when they come; they're perfect chances to build some extra exercise into your day.

We mean actual exercises—the Stealth Exercises described on page 120. Do them while standing in line at the bank, sitting in traffic, or cooling your heels while waiting at the assigned time and place for friends or family members (who apparently don't know how to tell time). Others you can do in the privacy of your home while you go about everyday activities, such as brushing your teeth or heating a pot of water for tea.

STEP THREE

Make Active Fun Your First Choice

At a neighborhood picnic, are you the person with their hands in the chips and deviled eggs, or is your hand in a baseball glove, attempting to defend third base? At the park, are you the parent in the thick of the Frisbee game or climbing the monkey bars or the one huddled on the park bench looking bored? We promise: You don't have to be fit, fast, or good at sports to get out there and have some fun.

Play with kids. Impromptu games of basketball, touch football, or tag or just jumping rope or throwing a ball will help you use energy and set a good example of active play for the children. This kind of play can burn 80 to 137 calories every 10 minutes.

See exercise as a new social opportunity. Use your desire to get more physical activity as your motivation to sign up for a tango class, biking club, or Pilates lesson—something you've always wanted to try or something you never thought you'd do. Making new friends will be an added bonus—and the opportunity to see them will serve as motivation to show up.

Make it a family event. Set up a badminton net or softball diamond in your backyard and get a game going with your family (and neighbors if you need more players). And opt for active family fun such as water parks, sledding hills, playgrounds, pools, and zoos.

Join a sports team. Most communities have soccer, baseball, softball, and even basketball teams for, ahem, older athletes. If you want a little less intensity, try coaching a kids team or even refereeing. It will keep you on your feet.

Try yoga. In addition to reducing stress, research indicates that regular yoga practice can help lower blood sugar as well as improve weight, blood pressure, and cholesterol levels.

Go bowling instead of going out for ice cream. You'll burn 100 calories in just a half hour. Haven't bowled in decades? Ask to have the bumpers put up along the sides of the lane; it'll improve your score and make the game more fun.

Join a hiking club or download a map, grab a friend and go exploring. If you love wandering in nature, pick a park, mountain, beach, or lake that's close by. Find a map, and check if there's an admission fee. Also consider cultivating an interest in birds. Bird-watching is one of America's hottest hobbies, thanks to the wonderful diversity of colors, shapes, songs, and personalities among North American birds.

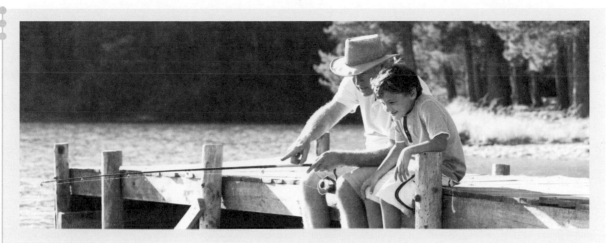

15 Ways to Burn 100 Calories

Whether you're trying to lose weight or maintain a healthy weight, it's important to not get overwhelmed by the big picture—"I have to lose 20 pounds"—but, instead, to focus on the little, everyday things that can make a big difference. For instance, if you burn an extra 100 calories a day, even if you don't change your eating habits at all, you'll lose about 10.5 pounds over the course of a year. What's it take to burn 100 calories? Not much.*

1. Go roller-skating. In just 12 minutes (assuming you haven't broken your arm) you've burned off 100 calories.

2. Go grocery shopping. A 38-minute grocery shopping trip burns 100 calories; you'll burn another 100 calories carrying the groceries to your car and then into your house.

3. Play Frisbee. Half an hour is all it takes—and that assumes you're not doing a lot of running after wild throws.

4. Put up a Christmas tree. Forty minutes of stringing lights and hanging ornaments is all that's needed to burn 100 calories and decorate for the holidays. If you don't celebrate, help a friend who does!

5. Usher for your church, temple, or synagogue. After 45 minutes, you'll have not only greeted all the parishioners but will also have burned 100 calories.

6. Make dinner. Pick one that requires chopping. If it takes you 35 minutes to get dinner ready, you've just burned your 100.

7. Jump rope. Even slow jumping burns 100 calories in 11 minutes; jump faster, and it takes only about 7 minutes.

8. Clean out your garage. Put in half an hour of sorting. By then, you'll have cleared at least one small space and burned 100 calories.

9. Jog in place for 11 minutes. Do it during the commercials of a 30-minute TV show.

10. Dance the flamenco. Just 15 minutes of fast ballroom dancing will do it.

11. Walk a dog. In half an hour, you'll have burned 100 calories, and he'll have stretched all four legs and sniffed to his heart's content. If you don't have a dog, offer to walk your neighbor's dog!

12. Iron your clothes. Do it for 40 minutes.

13. Hit the driving range for 30 minutes. You'll improve your golf game and burn 100 calories.

14. Play golf. Carry your clubs and walk the course, and you'll burn 100 calories every 20 minutes.

15. Go fishing. It's peaceful and stress-free, and 30 minutes of it burns about 100 calories.

*All estimates based on a 150-pound, 42-year-old woman.

The *Reverse Diabetes* Stealth Exercises

Tree Pose

You can do this variation of a yoga move while combing your hair or brushing your teeth.

Stand up straight with your legs together. Slowly raise your right knee to the side, resting the bottom of your right foot against the inner calf of your left leg. Balance there for a count of 15, keeping your left knee unlocked. Pull in your stomach for support and keep your back straight and your chin up. Repeat on the other side.

BENEFIT Strengthens the lower body and core support muscles of the lower back and abdomen.

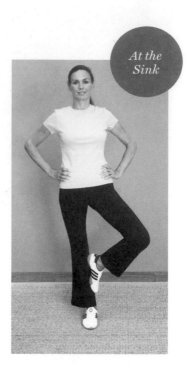

At the Sink

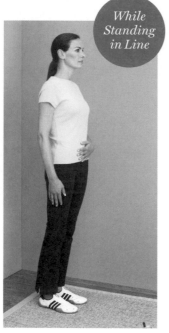

While Standing in Line

Standing Ab Squeeze

Keeping your neck, shoulders, and arms relaxed, pull in and tighten the muscles of your abdomen. (Picture a belt being tightened around your midsection.) Hold for 30 seconds, breathing as normally as possible. Do this three times.

BENEFIT Doing this exercise while standing strengthens muscles that support your back against the strain of extra weight in your gut.

Butt Buster

Stand up straight with your feet hip-width apart. Squeeze the muscles of your buttocks together as tightly as you can, hold in your stomach, and move your right leg about 2 inches behind you with your foot off the floor. Hold for 10 seconds, then switch legs.

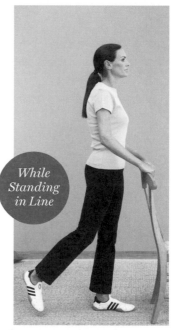

While Standing in Line

BENEFIT Strengthens the humble but powerful muscles in your rear, which are involved in virtually every movement your body makes.

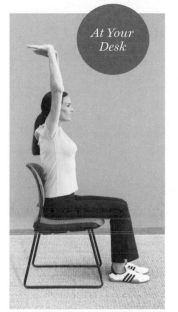

At Your Desk

Overhead Press

Sit up straight with your back firmly against the back of your chair and your feet flat on the floor, about hip-width apart. Raise your arms over your head with your palms flat and your elbows facing to the sides. Inhale and press up as if you were going to push the ceiling with your hands. Hold for 30 seconds, breathing normally. Repeat.

BENEFIT The palm position of this exercise isolates and strengthens the muscles of the shoulders.

Thigh Toner

Sit up straight. While tucking in your stomach muscles, curl your hands into fists and place them between your knees. Squeeze your fists with your thighs and hold for 30 seconds. Repeat.

BENEFIT Strengthens and firms the difficult-to-isolate muscles of the inner thighs.

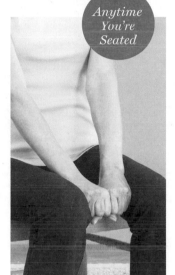

Anytime You're Seated

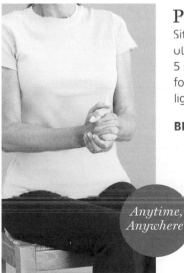

Palm Clasp

Sit up straight and grab one hand with the other. Press your palms together hard for 5 seconds, then release. Do this movement four times. You can also do this one at red lights or while watching TV.

BENEFIT Strengthens the chest and arms.

Anytime, Anywhere

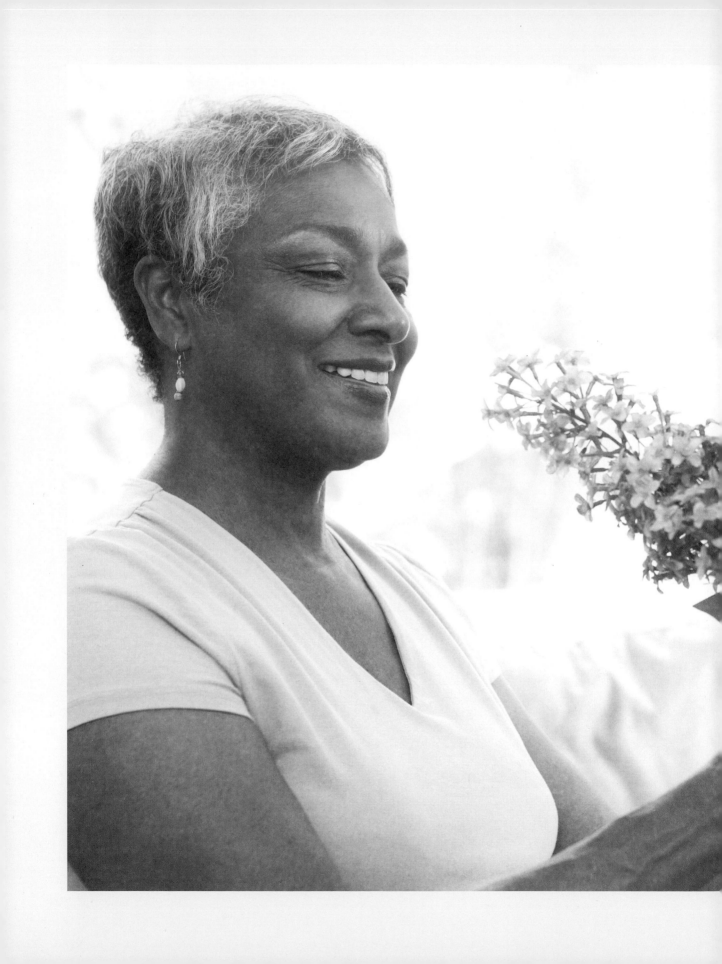

3

CHOOSE
to Reverse Diabetes

- Inspire Change
- Plan Ahead
- Rest and Recharge

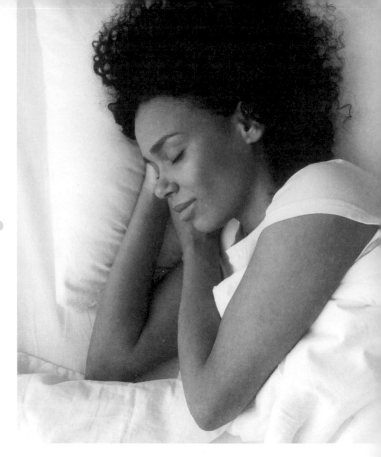

The Plan

Your Eat and Move goals won't happen automatically. You must consciously choose to put in the work day after day. Some days that will be easy. Other days, you'll need some support—and that's where your Choose Plan comes in. These motivational, sleep, and stress management strategies lay the foundation for long-term change.

What to Do

GOAL 1
Practice the subtle art of self-motivation

Reversing diabetes begins in your mind—by unlocking the motivational rocket fuel needed for lasting change. By keeping your deepest reasons for change front and center, you'll be more prepared to face the day-to-day challenges of managing your blood sugar and lifestyle. Strong motivation has been linked to improved blood sugar as well as fewer diabetes complications.

GOAL 2
Sleep restfully

Think of how you feel after a great night's sleep. With the strategies in this section, you'll be able to have that kind of all-day energy more often, giving you the mental clarity you need to create new eating and movement habits. On top of that, getting enough deep, restful sleep serves as a powerful metabolic balm that can help you control blood sugar, feel less hungry between meals, and lose weight more easily.

GOAL 3
Embrace self-care

Indulging in "me" time—as well as using it to melt away tension—isn't a luxury. It's a necessity, especially for blood sugar control, maintaining a healthy weight, and staying on track with healthy lifestyle changes. We'll introduce you to a wide range of activities to choose from, so you can create the ultimate self-care routine for *you*.

What to Record

1. HOW MUCH SLEEP YOU GOT LAST NIGHT

For each day of your 12-week challenge, record the number of hours you sleep using the habit trackers beginning on page 146. Aim for seven to eight hours, and notice how you're feeling if you get more or less. You'll see how your sleep affects your blood sugar and your success with healthy eating and exercise.

2. WHETHER YOU MADE TIME FOR SELF-CARE

It's every bit as important to your health as eating well and exercising. In your habit tracker, check your self-care box whenever you do something just for you. That might be as simple as coffee with a friend or signing up for a massage or meditation class.

3. HOW YOU FEEL

Was it an excellent or pretty good day, or are you glad that you'll get a fresh start tomorrow? Rating your attitude every day is a great reminder that attitude counts—and an opportunity for an honest self-evaluation of your outlook. Paying attention to your attitude can help you cultivate the art of supporting your own best efforts—another powerful tool for great diabetes self-care. In your habit tracker, you'll find emojis to circle to indicate how you feel.

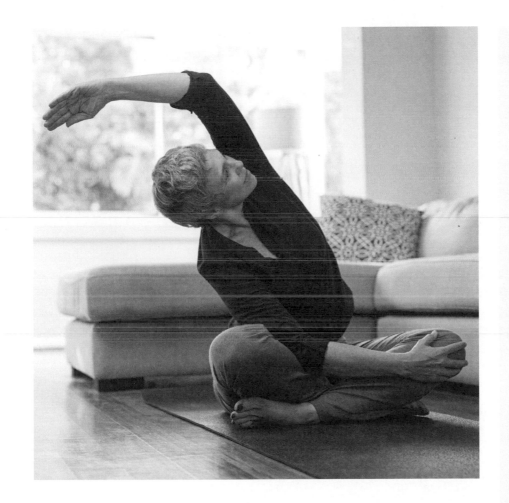

Before You Begin

Take the quiz on page 126.

This quiz will help you assess whether your sleep habits, mind-set, and self-care skills are helping you manage your diabetes—or getting in the way of your success. As always, answer as frankly as possible, and take your results seriously: They'll tell you in which areas of your life you'll want to make some changes in order to choose to reverse diabetes. If the results hint at burnout or a serious sleep problem such as insomnia or sleep apnea, it warrants a visit to your doctor.

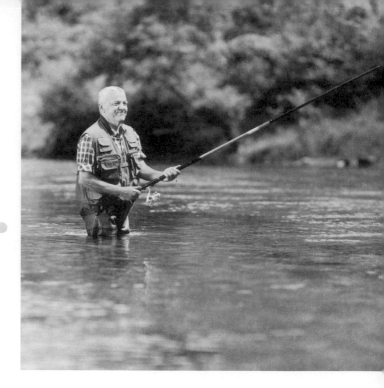

The Quiz

Are you making the everyday choices that add up to consistently healthy eating and movement habits? Or are stress, low motivation, depression, or lack of sleep standing between you and the change you'd like to accomplish? Take our quiz and find out.

Scan to take this quiz online.

1. On a typical weeknight I:
 a. Stay up late paying bills, surfing the Internet, or watching TV.
 b. Try my best to hit the hay in time for seven to eight hours of sleep.
 c. Dread the bed, knowing I'll lay awake for hours.

2. In the morning I:
 a. Usually wish I'd gone to bed earlier the night before.
 b. Feel pretty good.
 c. Am exhausted.

3. During the night I:
 a. Often wake up and can't get back to sleep.
 b. Sleep like a baby.
 c. Snore so loudly my spouse or partner has to nudge me.

4. I would say my sleep quality is:
 a. Not up to par because I'm doing the wrong things.
 b. Good or great.
 c. Poor despite my best efforts.

5. My motivation for controlling my blood sugar is:
 a. Starting to slip; keeping up with diabetes is becoming more difficult.
 b. Going strong.
 c. Nearly gone; I feel overwhelmed and tired of all this work.

6. In the past two weeks I've felt:
 a. Somewhat tense, irritated, or stressed out.
 b. Pretty good—I'm weathering difficult days and good days equally well.
 c. Down, depressed, or not interested in the things that I usually enjoy.

7. When someone cuts me off in traffic or something else stressful happens, I:
 a. Fume for a little while, then get over it.
 b. Feel a brief jolt of frustration, then forget about it.
 c. Become extremely angry and stay that way.

8. **At the end of the day I:**
   a. Overeat, have several alcoholic drinks, or watch a lot of TV to drown out the stress.
   b. Spend some time unwinding in my favorite way.
   c. Replay the day's stresses over and over in my mind, or face new ones at home. There's no downtime.

9. **When I get off course with managing my diabetes—by overeating, skipping exercise, or not testing my blood sugar enough—I tend to:**
   a. Feel guilty—but vow to do better.
   b. Remind myself that ups and downs are normal, and I can make a fresh start tomorrow.
   c. Feel defeated and make even more mistakes.

Your Score

Give yourself 1 point for each "a" you circled, 2 points for each "b" answer, and 0 points for each "c."

15–18 points
You're choosing to reverse your diabetes.
You're taking pretty good care of yourself by getting enough sleep, keeping a positive attitude, and controlling stress. But unless you scored a perfect 18, there's always room for improvement!

10–14 points
You're short-changing yourself a bit.
Giving higher priority to quality sleep and quality leisure time can help you get a better handle on your blood sugar and stave off stress. Using motivational strategies will help you to keep up the healthy lifestyle you desire.

0–9 points
You have some room for improvement—but don't stress or beat yourself up over it.
The 12-week challenge was made for you. You'll start slowly, at a pace you can manage. By the end, retake this and other quizzes so you can feel great about how much you've improved.

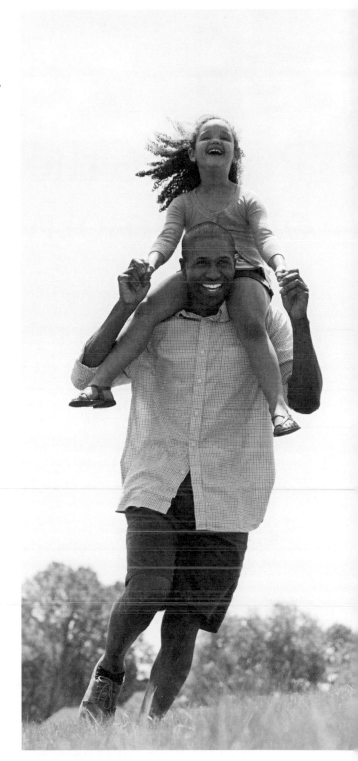

GOAL 1

Practice the subtle art of self-motivation

WE OFTEN ASSUME THAT, if we want something badly enough, our willpower will take care of itself. In other words, we think we can tell ourselves "just do it!" and everything will get done.

Here's a question to deeply consider: *How has "just do it!" worked for you in the past?*

If you're like most people, the answer is: Not so much.

Without continually stocking your motivational fire, inspiration usually wanes somewhere around the halfway mark, finds research from New York University. This happens for two reasons:

You no longer remember how you felt in the beginning. All of those reasons that once fired you up now seem distant. At the same time, the end is still far enough away that it seems unreachable.

Humans tend to put a greater value on short-term, smaller rewards in the present (let's walk to the fridge and see if something fun is inside) over long-term bigger rewards in the future (if I don't eat this donut, I'll be healthier later on). This psychological phenomenon (called "delay discounting") most likely kept humans alive during hunting and gathering times. In other words, the puny antelope our ancient ancestor could see was more likely to stop starvation than the herd of antelope that might have been on the other side of a far away hill.

Thankfully, researchers have uncovered powerful ways to overcome motivational slumps, allowing you to choose to reverse diabetes consistently.

STEP ONE
Keep Your Past Close

Spend time answering these questions:

- Why do you want to reverse diabetes?
- Why do you want to lose weight?
- Why do you want to get healthier?

Maybe you're reading this and thinking "well, duh." We challenge you: Dig deeper than that.

"Be healthy" and "weigh less" are fuzzy goals. They're the kind of goals that fall into the "it'd be nice if" category rather than the "I am absolutely making this happen" category.

To motivate yourself over the hump, you want a specific and very personal goal.

So, again: Why do you want to reverse diabetes?

If you draw a blank, turn the question around and consider the reverse: Why don't you want to allow diabetes to run its course? Why don't you want to be unhealthy? What scares you about the idea of staying the same?

Get crystal clear about those fears. Maybe you're afraid that you won't be able to be there for your spouse or partner, children, or grandchildren. Maybe you're frustrated about not having enough energy to get through the workday—and you're afraid you're going to lose your job over it.

Find the reason that almost compels you to get up and munch on a stalk of broccoli.

Then, come up with a way to keep your reason close, so that your starting point never feels distant. Maybe you:

- Write a postcard or letter to yourself to read everyday, reminding you of the reasons you are doing this.

- Record a video of yourself giving a motivational pep talk to the future you who is starting to wonder, "What's the point?"

STEP TWO

Bring Your Future Into Your Present

When humans visualize their future selves, they're able to continually motivate themselves over the long term, researchers have found. For example, when people with type 2 diabetes imagined themselves taking their medications regularly in the future, they improved how regularly they followed their medication regimen.

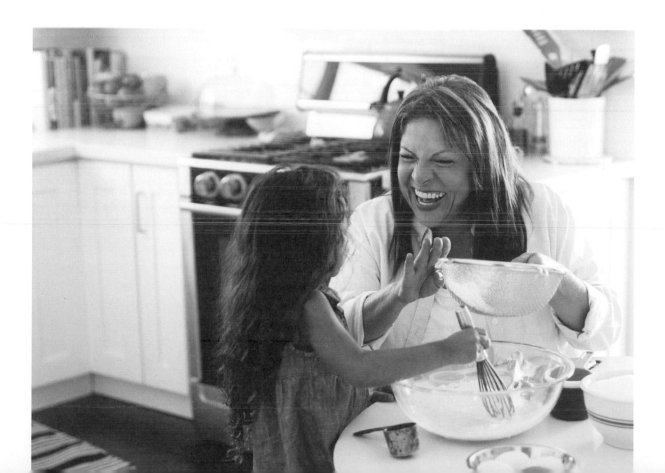

There are a few ways to do this.

- Imagine your ideal future self. Imagine the person who loves to walk, strength train, and eat veggies.

- See yourself doing the tasks you want to get done—and imagine every single step of the process. If you want to go to the gym regularly, for example, see yourself hopping out of bed, getting dressed, grabbing your gym bag, and so on.

- Consider the future you fear. What future will likely unfold if you don't eat your veggies or walk regularly? Try to make it as real as possible by using all of your senses.

STEP THREE

Brainstorm Ways to Make Change Nonnegotiable

Let's say you wanted to get up everyday at six in the morning to fit in a walk. You could set an alarm, but alarms are easy to turn off and ignore. So what else might you do?

Well, maybe you set a second alarm that is far enough away from your bed that you can't turn it off without actually getting up. But you could turn off that one and just crawl back into bed, right?

So—what else?

What about walking with someone else—someone who will ring your doorbell and wake your whole family if you are not outside by 6:05 a.m.?

Now that just might work.

Use this thought process for other tasks that you want to make non-negotiable. Consider:

- How can you make this task easier for yourself to do regularly?

- How can you make skipping the task harder for yourself?

STEP FOUR

Link New Tasks to Established Routines

Chances are, you do dozens of things every day without even thinking about them. We're talking about things such as brushing your teeth, making coffee, and showering. These activities are automated—and they can serve as the foundation for habit formation.

When you stack a new action (say, taking your medicine) onto an existing habit (say, brushing your teeth), you increase the likelihood of getting both tasks done.

Consider the many activities you do every day and how you might stack a new habit right before, during, or after it. Maybe you…

- Do a set of wall push ups while waiting for your coffee to drip.

- Stretch whenever you watch your favorite TV show.

- Go for a walk just after washing the dishes.

STEP FIVE

Line Up Coaches and Cheerleaders

Changing your lifestyle requires work—and you don't need to do all of it alone. Think about who might be able to ease this journey for you. And conversely, who might make it harder?

Once you have those answers, talk to family members, friends, and coworkers about how they can help you. Maybe you join a coworker everyday at lunch for a walk. Perhaps your partner doesn't mind helping you search for healthy recipes. And your kids or grandkids might love celebrating with you when you accomplish specific goals.

GOAL **2**

Sleep restfully

SLEEP PROBLEMS ARE deeply connected with insulin resistance, high blood sugar, and hormone changes that lead to weight gain. And it's a vicious circle: unstable blood sugar leads to disturbed sleep, which leads to unstable blood sugar.

Sleep and body fat also interact in a similarly vicious circle. Lack of sleep leads to elevations in the hunger hormone ghrelin, which can increase cravings for sugar and starchy carbs. That, in turn, can lead to unstable blood sugar, which leads to disturbed sleep. Gain enough weight and sleep apnea can develop, raising the risk for developing diabetes and heart problems, too.

On the bright side, healthy habits can form a virtuous circle. Exercise, for example, tends to improve sleep—and improved sleep gives you more energy for exercise. Improving your sleep is one of those cornerstone habits that can make every other lifestyle change a heck of a lot easier. Here's how to set yourself up for deep, restful slumber.

STEP ONE
Make Your Mornings Brighter

Wake up at the same time every morning. This is one of the surest ways to train your body to fall asleep at the same time every night.

Important: For best results, you'll want to follow your wake routine on the weekends as well as during the week.

Bathe yourself in morning sunlight. Morning light exposure does more to jolt you awake. It also helps to set your brain's sleep-wake clock, causing you to feel drowsy hours later when it's time to crawl into bed. Here's a hint that will save you money: Outdoor sunlight—even on a cloudy day—is thousands of lux brighter than the typical light machine you might purchase.

You only need about 5 to 10 minutes to do the trick.

STEP TWO
Make Sleep-Friendly Choices Throughout the Day

Cut back on caffeine. Caffeine blocks the action of a sleep-inducing brain chemical called adenosine. It takes three to seven hours for your body to metabolize just half the caffeine in a cup of tea or coffee. If you can't live without it, relegate your caffeine to the morning and consider switching to half caf, half decaf. Or switch to green tea, which has less caffeine and many other health benefits.

131

Move every day. Physical activity improves sleep as effectively as powerful sleeping pills called benzodiazepines, finds research. Consider pairing your morning sunlight exposure with a walk to fully benefit.

Allow at least three hours between dinner and bedtime. The brain does not sleep well on a full stomach. If you know that you have a busy day planned the following day, have your big meal at lunchtime and a lighter meal as early as possible in the evening.

However, some people may need a snack close to bedtime for better blood glucose management. If you find you are still hungry before bedtime, avoid sugar; try a small handful of nuts. Talk with your registered dietitian or certified diabetes educator for individualized guidance.

STEP THREE
Create a Bedtime Routine

Power down in the hours before bed. Turn down overhead lighting. Stay away from agitating activities such as watching heart-pounding horror movies or checking anger-producing social media accounts. Turn off your computer and put your phone on silent mode.

Sugar Buster Quiz

Q: Nap or no nap?
A: It depends on *how* you nap.

Naps can be restorative as long as they are shorter than 30 minutes and taken late morning or early afternoon. Nap later in the day or longer than 30 minutes and you risk tossing and turning later in the evening.

If You Need Professional Help

If you've tried all of the sleep advice from this chapter and you're still tossing and turning, you might benefit from sessions with a therapist trained in Cognitive Behavioral Therapy for Insomnia (CBT-I). This type of therapy helps you to identify and address the thoughts, feelings, and behaviors that contribute to your sleep problems. It usually takes six to eight sessions to see noticeable sleep improvements.

Signal to yourself that it's time to sleep. By going through the same motions night after night, you'll train your body to feel sleepy. Maybe you take a bath or shower, change into jammies, read quietly, or do a little relaxing yoga

Slumber in a sleep sanctuary. Organize your bedroom so that it invites you to crawl into bed. Consider decorating it in soothing colors, using pleasing scents (such as lavender), and getting in the habit of keeping it neat and tidy. Lowering your home's temperature in the evening can also help signal to your body that it's time to sleep, experts say. You may also find that you sleep better in the dark. If your eyelids flutter open as you move from one stage of sleep to another, even streetlights or a full moon can wake you.

Soothe yourself with sound. Remember when you were little and your mom's voice singing a lullaby never failed to put you to sleep? Numerous devices and apps today can help recreate the effect with calming music, relaxing meditations, white noise, and even bedtime stories for adults.

Improving sleep makes every other lifestyle change easier.

STEP FOUR

Troubleshoot Sleep Issues

Keep a worry book. Put a small journal and a pen on your bedside table. Before switching off the light, use it to jot down any worrisome thoughts or tasks for the following day. Then close the book, put it on your night stand, turn out the light, and go to sleep.

Get up if you're not sleeping. Letting yourself toss and turn at night to the point of frustration creates anxiety about sleep that can make insomnia worse. If you wake at two in the morning, get up to go read a book or magazine in the living room, do a few stretches, or try one of the self-care strategies from the next section. Don't go back to bed until you feel sleepy enough to fall asleep.

GOAL 3

Embrace self-care

YOU KNOW FIRSTHAND all about your body's responses to stress—the way you feel keyed-up or angry and how your head starts to throb, your armpits start to sweat, or your neck muscles tense up.

You may be less familiar with your body's relaxation response—an innate, natural ability each of us has to enter into a physical state of thorough, sweet relaxation. It's that deep-down *ahhhh* you may notice when you hold hands with your spouse or partner, hug a child, hold a sleeping baby, watch the ocean waves, listen to soothing music, or engage in prayer or meditation. Believe it or not, you can teach yourself to elicit this relaxation response whenever you like, with a little practice. Here's how to get there.

STEP ONE

Breathe Deeply, Especially Before Meals

When we're calm, we naturally take slow, deep breaths. When we're frantic, on the other hand, our breathing becomes shallow, almost as if the air remains caught in our throat.

Interestingly, by mimicking how our bodies breathe when relaxed, we can bring about a relaxed mental state. In other words, by faking calm (by breathing deeply) you end up truly feeling calm. But it's easy to forget to do it.

That's why we recommend using advice you learned in Goal 1: Habit stacking. By stacking the new habit of deep breathing with something you already do everyday, you'll be more likely to breathe deeply on a regular basis.

A great place to slip in some deep breathing: just before eating. You eat every day, several times a day, giving you plenty of opportunities to breathe. As a side benefit, deep breathing will likely help you eat more slowly and mindfully, helping you to feel more satisfied on smaller portions.

To do it, pause before digging into your meal. Place a hand on your tummy to remind yourself to breathe deeply. Then inhale as if you are smelling a flower. Exhale through your mouth as if you are blowing out a candle. Repeat two to three times.

STEP TWO

Slow Down at the Table

Turn meal time into "me" time. Rather than rush through your meals or try to multitask while eating, turn off the TV, put down your phone, and see if you can slow down and truly savor the experience. Imagine that you're having this meal

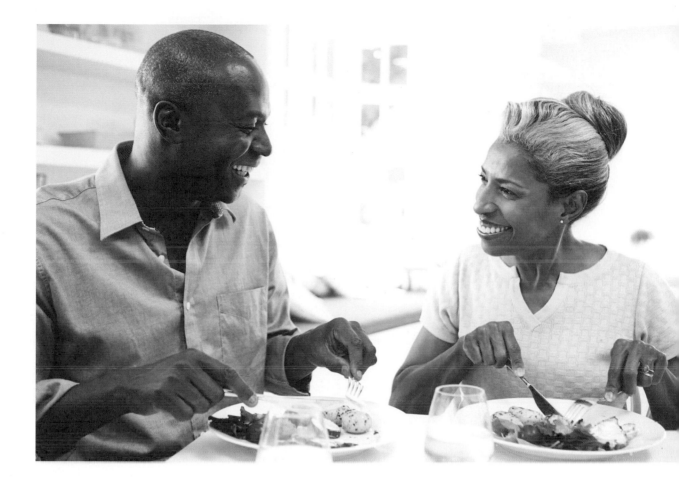

during an expensive vacation and you want to get the most out of it.

Slow, mindful eating offers real benefits, far beyond giving you an oasis of calm in your day. It can also help you to automatically eat less overall. When study participants took 24 minutes to consume a meal, they felt fuller after the meal and automatically ate less later in the day than did people who consumed the same meal in just six minutes.

Even better, enjoy your meal with your family or friends. Connecting with people you love can be a wonderful form of self-care and is demonstrated to have numerous health benefits.

STEP THREE
Think About Others

Say thank you more often. Gratitude can help you dial down negative, self-focused thinking. In fact, when depressed college students wrote a letter of gratitude to another person each week for three weeks, their mental health improved more over 12 weeks than another group of college students who received typical counseling.

Be generous. Studies consistently show that giving time—to a friend, a charity, or a stranger—makes people feel less time-starved. It can also fuel you with a sense of meaning and purpose.

135

STEP FOUR
Explore Self-Compassion

Though the words "self-compassion" might sound woo-woo, this established psychological technique is grounded in research, with studies showing that it can reduce your risk of heart disease.

Developed by Kristin Neff, PhD, an associate professor at the University of Texas at Austin, it involves three elements: self kindness, connecting with common humanity and mindfulness. To try it:

1. Consider a situation where you feel threatened.

2. Sit or stand tall, in a confident posture.

3. See if you can acknowledge the harm without fixating on the person who did the harm. You might say to yourself, "This isn't fair" or "I don't like being treated like this."

4. Now link your experience to the experience of others. Maybe you tell yourself, "This has happened to other people too."

5. Place your fist over your heart as you commit to standing up for yourself. Maybe you say, "I will speak up for myself."

6. Place your remaining hand over your fist. Hold it with kindness and consider: How will you use your fierce self-compassion to take action?

STEP FIVE
Experiment With Mindfulness

A form of meditation, mindfulness can help you improve how you manage your diabetes, according to a study on veterans who participated in the Mind-STRIDE program (Mindful Stress Reduction In Diabetes Education). After three months of mindfulness training, on average, the veterans' A1C levels fell from 8.3 to 7.3, and their diabetes management improved.

You can practice it anywhere, simply by bringing your attention to your thoughts, feelings, and sensations. If you are washing the dishes, for example, notice how the warm water and soap feels on your hands. Take note of thoughts about washing the dishes, such as "Dang it, why am I always the one stuck doing this?" Do the same with your feelings about the activity.

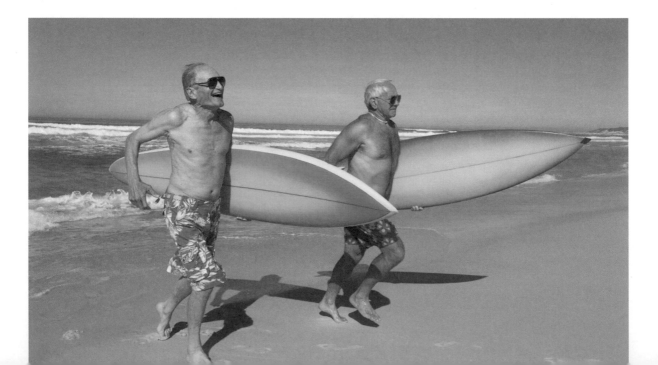

That awareness—of thoughts, feelings, and sensations—is mindfulness.

Go Outside

Exposure to nature has been linked to a reduced risk of everything from type 2 diabetes to cardiovascular disease to premature death. And the definition of nature is pretty broad. In studies, everything from vast undeveloped landscapes to urban parks helped people to feel calmer.

Use Movement to Relax

One of the most effective ways to defuse stress is to run away from it—or at least walk briskly. In one study that asked 38 men and 35 women to keep diaries of their activity, mood, and stress, volunteers reported that they felt less anxious on days when they were physically active than on days when they didn't exercise. Even when stressful events occurred, people in the study said they felt less troubled on their physically active days.

Turn your workouts into stress reducers. Virtually any kind of physical activity seems to relieve stress, although some researchers think that activities that involve repetitive movements—walking, running, cycling, or swimming, for instance—may offer the best defense. Many people consider swimming to be one of the most relaxing exercises, a soothing way to literally go with the flow. Repeating a physical movement over and over again somehow seems to ease mind and body.

Think about some ways to make your workout even more relaxing. If you're a walker, be aware of the way your arms swing from front to back and the rhythm of your gait. Repeat a soothing word or phrase each time you exhale. If you work out on an exercise cycle or stair machine at a fitness club, ignore what's on the big TV screen in the room. Scientists have found that watching television makes people more jittery, not less. If you can't turn off the TV, look elsewhere and focus on your breathing, or plug yourself into some soothing music.

Discover yoga. Looking for a simple way to relax, refresh your energy, become more limber, and strengthen muscles at the same time? Yoga may be just the ticket. Exercise scientists have long known that yoga offers a great way to stretch, increase strength, and improve balance. Now psychologists are discovering that it can also ease a troubled mind. At Oxford University, a researcher divided 71 people into three groups. One group practiced simple relaxation techniques such as deep breathing. The second group visualized themselves feeling less tense. The third did a half-hour yoga routine.

The relaxers and the visualizers felt sluggish afterward. The people in the yoga group reported feeling more energetic and emotionally content after their class.

How to get started? Several of the stretches you'll find in this section are based on yoga positions. If you find that you like doing these stretches, you may want to sign up for a yoga class online or at a local fitness center or yoga studio.

Establish a daily stretching routine. Stretching isn't just relaxing; it's also great for your whole body. Get in the habit of spending just 5 or 10 minutes stretching in the evenings, and you may find yourself sleeping better before you know it—and craving your stretches the next day. Try the stretches starting on the next page.

The *Reverse Diabetes* Stretching Routine

This series of 10 stretches takes just 5 to 10 minutes to complete and will make you feel as if a world-class massage therapist has just kneaded the tension out of every muscle in your body!

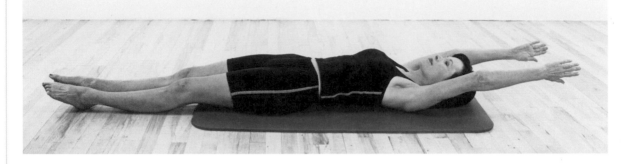

Lying Total Body Stretch

This stretch feels great and expands your whole body. It's particularly good for shoulders and abdominal muscles.

ONE Lie on your back with your legs extended and feet together or about hip-width apart.

TWO Extend your arms straight over your head and stretch your legs and toes, making your entire body as long as comfortably possible. Hold.

Smart Tip Take a deep breath before you begin the stretch, and exhale as you extend your hands and feet, then breathe normally as you hold, which enhances the stretch. Don't hold your breath; this prevents the abdominal muscles from relaxing.

Cross-Legged Seated Stretch

Sit up now for this soothing, classic back stretch, often used in yoga routines. It's great for lower back tension.

ONE Sit on the floor with your legs crossed and hands in front of you. Lean forward gently with your head down, rounding your back and "walking" your fingers forward until you feel a stretch in your lower and middle back. Hold.

TWO Walk your hands back to your legs and return to the starting position.

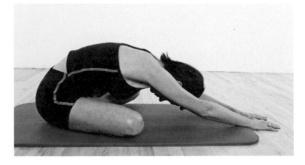

Smart Tip For a balanced stretch to both sides of the back, do this exercise twice, switching the leg that is crossed over the top of the other.

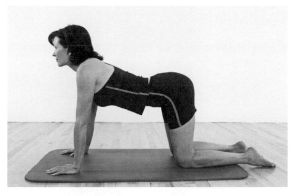

Cat Stretch

Pull yourself forward onto your hands and knees for another great stretch for your back.

ONE Get on your hands and knees. Tuck your chin toward your chest, and tighten your stomach muscles to arch your back. Hold.

TWO Relax, raising your head so you're looking straight ahead while letting your stomach drop toward the floor. Hold.

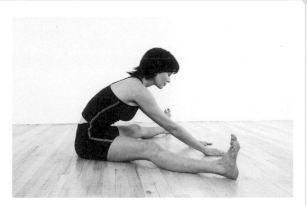

Seated V

This exercise lengthens the adductor muscles of the groin area in the inner thigh.

ONE Sit on the floor, back straight, legs extended, toes pointed toward the ceiling, and feet spread comfortably apart in a V.

TWO Keeping your back straight, gently "walk" your hands out in front of you until you feel a slight stretch in your inner thighs. Hold.

Smart Tip Use this position to stretch your hamstrings by putting your left hand on the inside of your right thigh and the right hand on the outside, then moving both hands down your leg. Hold. Repeat on the left leg.

Lying Pelvis Rotation

Relax onto the ground for this gentle torso stretch. It uses gravity to stretch the abductor muscles on the outside of the hip.

ONE Lie down on your right side, using your right arm as a pillow to support your head. Keeping your right leg straight, bend your left hip at a 90-degree angle so your knee is in front of you.

TWO Relax the muscles of your left leg so that your left knee slowly drops toward the ground. Stay relaxed and hold. Repeat with the other leg.

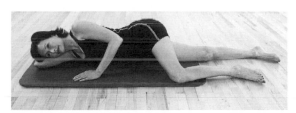

Smart Tip When you're more limber, try this variation: Lie down on your back with your knees bent and your feet flat on floor. Keeping your shoulders on the ground, slowly lower both knees to the right to get a stretch in left hip and buttocks. Hold; return to the starting position. Repeat on the other side.

continued >>>

Calf Stretch

Popular with runners, this stretch is ideal for anyone who walks a lot, as you're doing on the Move plan.

ONE Stand with toes of both feet about 12 to 18 inches from a wall.

TWO Supporting yourself against the wall with one or both hands, take a big step back with your right foot, keeping your left foot in place.

THREE Bending your left knee, keep your right leg straight with the heel flat on the ground to produce a gentle tug at the back of your lower leg. Hold; return to the starting position. Repeat on the other side.

Smart Tip Move your hips forward to increase the intensity of the stretch.

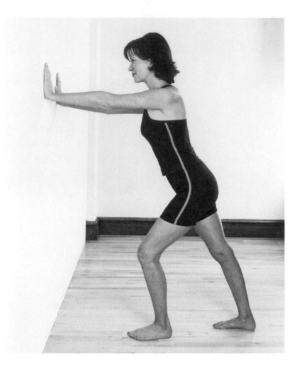

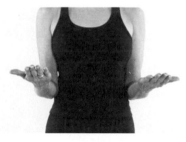

Forearm Flip

This stretch works muscles in your forearms that can hold tension after a day of typing or housework.

ONE Stand straight with your feet hip-width apart and knees slightly bent, arms hanging by your sides. Bend your elbows to 90 degrees with your palms facing upward as if you're holding a tray.

TWO Smoothly flip your hands over so the palms are facing the floor. Hold and return to the start position.

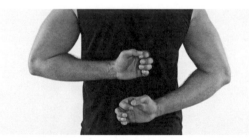

Knuckle Rub

Now it's on to your upper body to work out tension in your shoulder and neck muscles.

ONE Stand up straight with feet hip-width apart and knees slightly bent, hands down by your sides. Make a fist and, with knuckles facing forward, move your hands behind you and place them against your lower back.

TWO Gently move your knuckles up your back until you feel a stretch in the front part of your shoulder and your upper arms. Hold.

"Say Hello" Shoulder Stretch

Say hello to the world with this soothing shoulder stretch.

ONE Stand straight with your feet hip-width apart and knees slightly bent, arms hanging down and hands on the front part of the opposite thigh.

TWO Keeping your arms extended, lift your hands in a sideways and upward motion as high over your head as you can. Hold for one second and return to the starting position. Do six repetitions.

Smart Tip Breathe in as you slowly lift your arms, and exhale as you return; this helps you establish a rhythm and trains you to breathe more deeply.

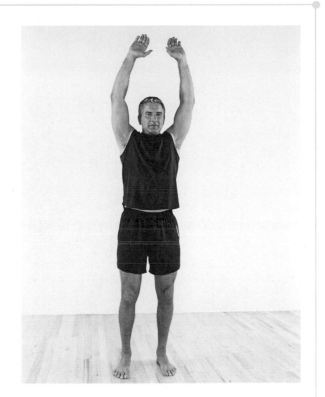

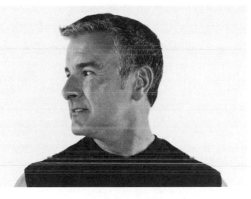

Neck Turn

If your neck is sensitive or in pain, do this exercise lying down to lessen the pressure.

ONE Sit or stand up straight with your eyes looking directly ahead.

TWO Slowly and smoothly move your head to the right side until you feel a slight stretch in the muscles on the opposite side of your neck. Relax and hold. Slowly return to the starting position and repeat on the other side.

Hold each stretch for 10 to 15 seconds. That's how long it usually takes for a muscle to relax and stay relaxed.

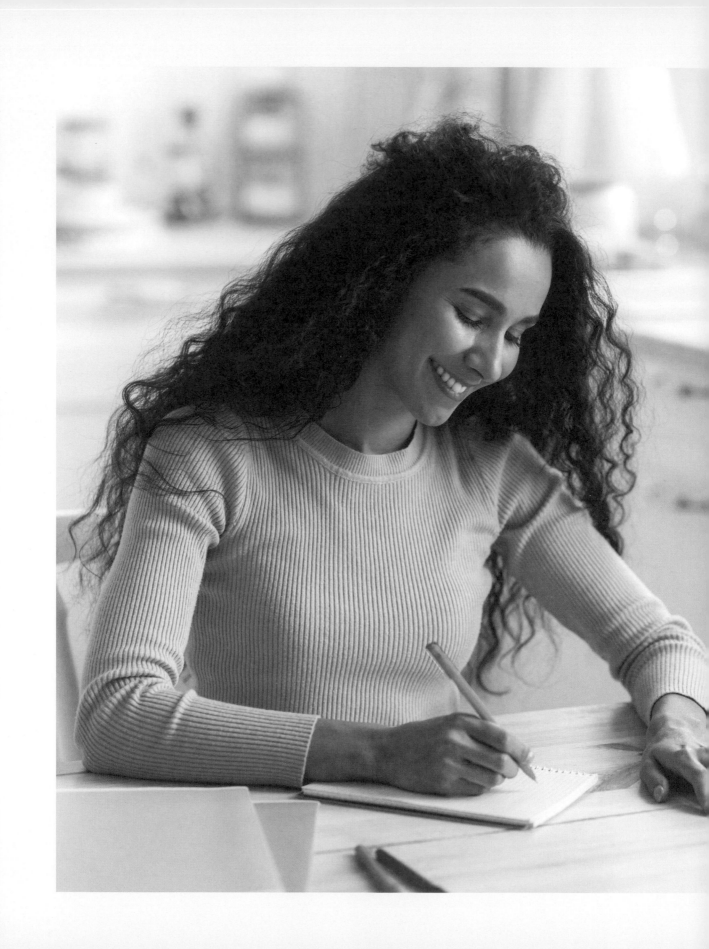

4

Reverse Diabetes
12-WEEK CHALLENGE

- Weekly Meal Planning
- Daily Progress Checks
- Successes and Confessions

Don't Let the Word "Challenge" Scare You

YES, YOU WILL ABSOLUTELY GROW in the next 12 weeks, taking on new goals and tasks. That said, we're going to ease you in, starting with practices that will feel reasonable and doable.

Then you'll build on those actions, one small step at a time, from one week to the next. By the end of the 12th week, you'll have mastered all of your Eat, Move, and Choose goals—and you'll see improvement in your blood sugar as well as the scale. For best results, use this advice.

Start where you are. The challenge begins with just noticing what you're eating and when you make time for self-care. Plus it calls for just 5 to 15 minutes of daily movement. If this suggested starting point seems too easy, feel free to adapt the instructions for your body, fitness level, and experience, with the goal of doing a little bit more than what you are doing today.

What counts as "a little bit more" varies from one person to another. For you, it might mean:

- Sneaking in an extra veggie serving each day
- Adding faster segments to your established 30-to-45-minute walks
- Taking five minutes to write in your gratitude journal.

Use the Reverse Diabetes habit tracker. Each week, you'll find a new checklist to track your progress. We recommend you either photocopy the ones from this book, create your own (using what we've provided as inspiration), or download them from thehealthy.com/reversediabetes/habittracker.

Scan to go to the checklists.

On each habit tracker, you'll find:

Space to take note of your weight or waist circumference. This is helpful to see fat loss progress from one week to another. If you feel uncomfortable using these methods, take notes on how your clothes fit (tight vs. roomy) or snap a weekly photo of yourself in the same outfit.

Space to record your blood sugar levels. Follow your health care provider's recommendations for testing your blood sugar. Based on your testing schedule, pick up to three daily readings to record in your habit tracker, such as first and last blood sugar result of the day and perhaps a reading right after you exercise or after your biggest meal. Over time, use your notes to notice whether these blood

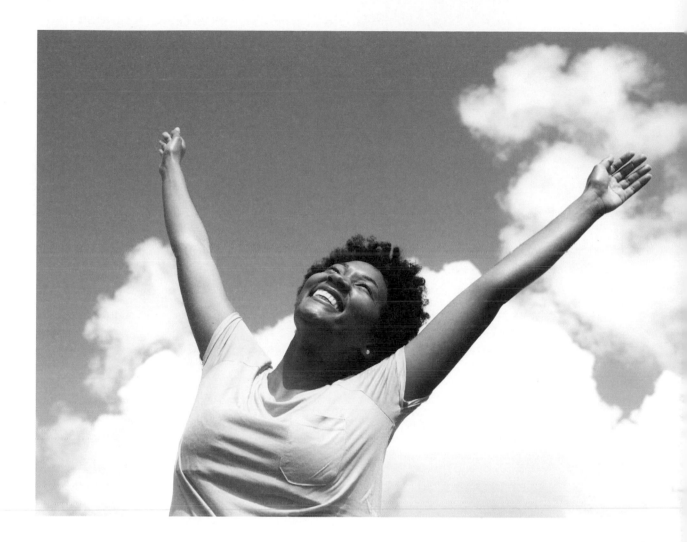

sugar levels have improved. If you are already logging your blood sugar with another method, there's no need to do additional tracking here.

A simple way to track your eating and exercise. Rather than writing down every single food you eat, the tracker will help you zero in on the presence (or absence) of smart foods. You will also jot down how many minutes you walk and anything else you do that's active.

An ultra simple self-care journal. Each day, circle the appropriate face to show how you feel.

As the weeks progress, you'll find more to track, including sleep, self-care, strength training, and more.

Celebrate your wins! Resist any urge to beat yourself up over unchecked boxes. Instead, try to get in the habit of looking for what you did right. Maybe you give yourself a pat on the back, mentally tell yourself "Yay you!" or pump your first in the air each time you check a box on the tracker. These small celebratory actions can help fuel motivation and consistency.

Week 1 Goals

EAT

Don't worry about changing what and how you eat this week. For now, we only want you to get in the habit of noticing what and how you eat (slowly, quickly, emotionally, or calmly).

Use your Reverse Diabetes habit tracker after each meal, checking off whether you had veggies, fruit, or protein. If you choose, you can also use the food diary on page 180 to track your eating habits in more detail.

Notice how long it takes you to eat and jot it down in your tracker.

Pay attention to why you eat. Were you physically hungry (empty, gnawing feeling in your stomach)? Then check the "hungry" box by that meal or snack. If you ate for a different reason (stress, craving/desire, mindlessly, peer pressure) jot it down in the notes area. This isn't about beating yourself up. Nor is it about trying to be perfect. Right now, you're just getting a baseline.

Use the Reverse Diabetes meal planner and shopping list templates (page 176-177). Check "planned" on your tracker for any meals you envisioned and shopped for ahead of time.

MOVE

Move everyday. It doesn't matter how far or how intensely you go. The important part is that you do something.

Pick a time of day to move. Maybe it's first thing in the morning, after lunch, or after dinner. See if you can get in the habit of walking for at least five minutes during your designated time slot.

Solve problems as they crop up. If you keep forgetting to walk—or if hurdles get in your way—don't beat yourself up over it. Instead, think about how you might overcome this challenge by asking yourself questions such as:

- "How might I make remembering to walk a little bit easier? What reminder system might help?"
- "How might I make prioritizing my walk a little bit easier? What needs to happen in order for me to get this walk in every day?"
- "What can I learn from this?"
- "How can I change my schedule in order to make a daily walk more likely?"
- "Who might I ask for help?"

Smart Tip When you go for your walk, seek soft surfaces. Walking or jogging on hard surfaces such as concrete can be hard on the joints and the feet. Whenever possible, walk on grass, a dirt road, or a running track at the local high school or YMCA.

CHOOSE

Use your habit tracker to take note of the time you go to bed, as well as the time you wake.

Check off your self-care box if you, for example, took a bath, practiced deep breathing, or otherwise did something just for you.

At the day's end, circle the emoji that best depicts how you feel.
☺ = happy
☹ = sad
😣 = angry
😴 = exhausted
☺ = neutral
😫 = anxious
😕 = determined

Habit Tracker

My numbers:
Weight or measurements: _____
Blood sugar (time/level): _____ / _____
_____ / _____
_____ / _____

EAT
Vegetables 0 1 2 3 4 5 6 7
Fruit 0 1 2 3
Smart protein 0 1 2 3

Breakfast: _____ minutes
□ Hungry □ Planned
Notes: _____

Lunch: _____ minutes
□ Hungry □ Planned
Notes: _____

Dinner: _____ minutes
□ Hungry □ Planned
Notes: _____

Snack: _____ minutes
□ Hungry □ Planned
Notes: _____

MOVE
□ Walked _____ minutes
□ Bonus movement _____

CHOOSE
Bedtime: _____
Wake time: _____
Self-care time: □ □ □ □ □

My attitude:
☺ ☹ 😣 😴 ☺ 😫 😕

147

Week 2 Goals

EAT

Take a look at your Week 1 checklists. On average, how many of your daily meals include a veggie, a protein, and/or a fruit? That's your baseline. You're going to build from there.

Consume one more daily veggie, fruit, and protein serving than you did last week. In other words, if you ate no veggies, on average, then your goal this week: One veggie every day.

If you had protein at breakfast, but not at any other meals, then your goal this week: Include protein at either lunch or dinner.

If you had two fruit servings most days, then your goal this week: Try to add a third.

Take a look at how long it took you to eat your meals last week, on average. See if you can make each meal last one or two minutes longer than the week before.

Plan at least two dinners ahead of time, using your Reverse Diabetes meal planner and grocery list builder in the Tools section.

MOVE

Walk five minutes longer than you did last week. In other words, if you walked five minutes most days last week, aim for at least 10 minutes a day this week.

CHOOSE

Take a look at your sleep and self-care practices from last week. Is there room for improvement? For sleep, for example, could you go to bed five minutes earlier than last week? For self-care, could your practice be more regular (most days instead of some)? Set a goal for yourself and write it down.

Smart Tip Make flavorful extra-virgin olive oil a part of your diet. A recent study showed that people who used small amounts of olive oil in salad dressings and vegetable dishes lost more weight and ate more vegetables than those who used nonfat dressings.

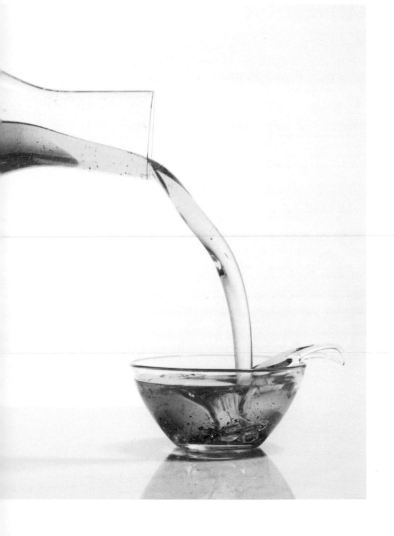

② Habit Tracker

My numbers:

Weight or measurements: _____

Blood sugar (time/level): _____ / _____

_____ / _____

_____ / _____

EAT

Vegetables 0 1 2 3 4 5 6 7
Fruit 0 1 2 3
Smart protein 0 1 2 3

Breakfast: _____ minutes
☐ Hungry ☐ Planned
Notes: _____

Lunch: _____ minutes
☐ Hungry ☐ Planned
Notes: _____

Dinner: _____ minutes
☐ Hungry ☐ Planned
Notes: _____

Snack: _____ minutes
☐ Hungry ☐ Planned
Notes: _____

MOVE

☐ Walked _____ minutes
☐ Bonus movement _____

CHOOSE

Bedtime: _____
Wake time: _____
Self-care time: ☐ ☐ ☐ ☐ ☐

My attitude:
☺ ☹ 😫 😴 😐 😁 😖

Week 3 Goals

EAT

Eat one additional daily veggie, protein, and fruit on top of what you had last week. In other words, if you ate one veggie, on average, last week, then your goal this week: Two veggies every day.

If you had protein at breakfast and lunch, then your goal this week: Include protein at dinner.

If you had three fruit servings most days, hooray! You've met this goal. Just try to remain consistent.

Make each meal last one or two minutes longer than the week before.

Plan at least three dinners ahead of time. Consider making a big meal on the weekend that you can use for a "leftover night" during the week.

NEW Wait until you feel stomach hungry (growling, empty sensation) before having any snacks. Remember: Don't beat yourself up if you eat for non-hunger reasons. Instead, celebrate the times you're able to triumphantly check the "hungry" box on your tracker.

MOVE

Make each daily walk five minutes longer than last week. So if you walked 15 minutes most days, then your goal is 20 minutes most days this week.

NEW Start doing Sugar Buster strength training routine. Do each sequence at least once during the week. It's okay to do fewer reps if needed.

CHOOSE

Take a look at your sleep and self-care practices from last week. Is there room for improvement? If so, set a goal based on what you see. That might be going to bed a little earlier, making your wake time more consistent, or adding a luxurious self-care practice on the weekend.

NEW Line up support. Ask a family member or friend to join you for some of your walks this week. Tell family and friends about your efforts to Reverse Diabetes and give them one way they can support and encourage you.

Smart Tip Exercise can cause blood sugar levels to rise or fall, so it's important to monitor your blood sugar before and after exercising. If your blood sugar is less than 100 mg/dl, have a snack, such as a piece of fruit, before you exercise. Don't exercise if your blood sugar level is less than 100 mg/dl.

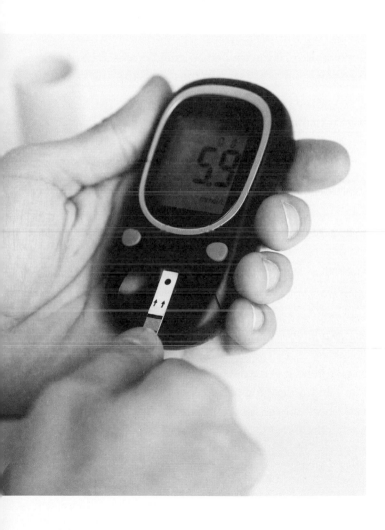

③ Habit Tracker

My numbers:

Weight or measurements: _____

Blood sugar (time/level): _____ / _____

_____ / _____

_____ / _____

EAT

Vegetables 0 1 2 3 4 5 6 7
Fruit 0 1 2 3
Smart protein 0 1 2 3

Breakfast: _____ minutes
☐ Hungry ☐ Planned
Notes: _____

Lunch: _____ minutes
☐ Hungry ☐ Planned
Notes: _____

Dinner: _____ minutes
☐ Hungry ☐ Planned
Notes: _____

Snack: _____ minutes
☐ Hungry ☐ Planned
Notes: _____

MOVE

☐ Walked _____ minutes
☐ Sugar Buster routine _____

CHOOSE

Bedtime: _____
Wake time: _____
Self-care time: ☐ ☐ ☐ ☐ ☐

My attitude:
☺ ☹ 😅 😴 😐 😁 😖

Week 4 Goals

EAT

Eat one more veggie, fruit, and smart protein daily than you did last week. In other words, if you ate two veggies, on average, then your goal this week: Three veggies every day. Same with fruit.

If you had protein at most meals some days, then your goal this week: Try to consume it more consistently—having it at most meals most days.

See if you can make each meal last one or two minutes longer than the week before. Chew each bite thoroughly before swallowing.

Try to plan at least four dinners ahead of time. Consider setting a theme to one or more weekly meals, whether it's taco night, burger night, or fish night. Then see if you can make that meal a bit healthier from one week to the next. For example, maybe burger night starts out with beef burger patties, a regular white flour bun, and Tater Tots. The week after, you might choose turkey burgers or a whole grain bun. The week after that, you might swap a salad for half of the Tots.

Continue to wait until you feel stomach hungry before snacking. See if you can improve on your progress from last week.

MOVE

Move five minutes longer daily than you did last week. So if you walked 20 minutes most days, then your goal is 25 minutes most days this week.

Keep doing the Sugar Busters strength training routine. Do each sequence at least once during the week.

CHOOSE

Take a look at your sleep and self-care practices from last week. Do you have room for improvement? If so, set a goal based on what you see.

NEW Breathe deeply before meals. Breathing through your nose, expanding your belly and filling your lungs from the bottom up. Exhale through your mouth, as if you're blowing out a candle. Try to take at least three deep breaths before your first bite—and notice how that affects how slowly you eat. Check off the "deep breathing" box once you complete this task.

Smart Tip Avoid all-or-nothing thinking. If you aim to exercise for 25 minutes but find you only have 10 minutes, don't feel that because you don't have time for your entire walk or workout you should do nothing. If all you have is 10 minutes, then exercise for 10 minutes.

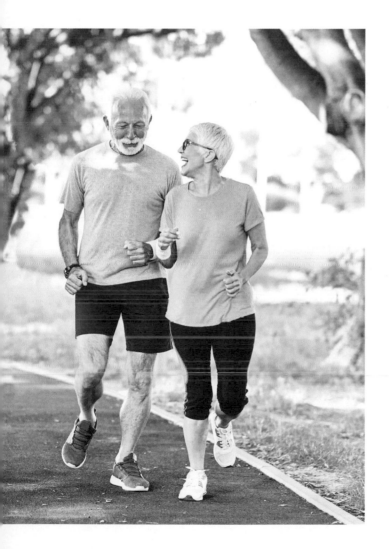

④ Habit Tracker

My numbers:
Weight or measurements: _____
Blood sugar (time/level): _____ / _____
_____ / _____
/

EAT
Vegetables 0 1 2 3 4 5 6 7
Fruit 0 1 2 3
Smart protein 0 1 2 3

Breakfast: _____ minutes
☐ Hungry ☐ Planned
Notes: _____

Lunch: _____ minutes
☐ Hungry ☐ Planned
Notes: _____

Dinner: _____ minutes
☐ Hungry ☐ Planned
Notes: _____

Snack: _____ minutes
☐ Hungry ☐ Planned
Notes: _____

MOVE
☐ Walked _____ minutes
☐ Sugar Buster routine _____

CHOOSE
Bedtime: _____
Wake time: _____
Self-care time: ☐ ☐ ☐ ☐
Deep breathing: ☐ ☐ ☐

My attitude:
☺ ☹ 😣 😓 ☺ 😁 😖

Week 5 Goals

EAT

Max out your veggie, protein, and fruit servings. Try to consume at least five veggie servings a day, three fruit servings a day, and protein with every meal.

NEW Smarten up at least one of your starch servings by opting for beans, lentils, potato (with the skin), whole grains, or another whole food instead of a highly-processed option.

NEW Start using the Reverse Diabetes plate (page 69) for portion control. As a refresher, half of your plate is veggies, a quarter is protein, and a quarter is starch. Devote up to one tablespoon (the size of your thumb) for good fats.

Make each meal last one or two minutes longer than the week before. Set a rule for yourself: You'll never put so much food in your mouth that you couldn't talk if you had to.

Plan at least five dinners ahead of time. It's okay if you plan to have one of these dinners out.

Continue to wait until you feel stomach hungry before snacking. See if you can improve on your progress from last week.

MOVE

Move five minutes longer than you did last week. So if you walked 25 minutes most days, then your goal is 30 minutes most days this week.

Keep doing the Sugar Busters strength training routine this week. Do each sequence at least once during the week.

NEW Add daily movement. In addition to your daily walks, look for other opportunities to move. Take the stairs, complete errands on foot, and take short movement breaks throughout the day.

CHOOSE

Continue to improve on sleep and self-care.

Continue to breathe deeply before meals.

NEW Develop a bedtime routine. At least 30 minutes before sleep time, start to wind down. Turn down your lights, flip off all electronics, and choose a soothing activity that helps nudge you into the mindset for sleep. Check the "bedtime routine" box whenever you complete this task.

Smart Tip For recipes that call for the smoky taste of bacon (soups, chowders, egg dishes, and bean dishes), choose lean turkey bacon instead of pork bacon. Even better, search online for a home-made tempeh, mushroom, or eggplant "bacon" recipe to try.

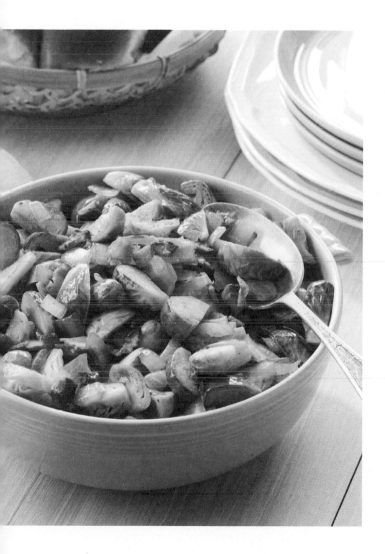

⑤ Habit Tracker

My numbers:

Weight or measurements: _____

Blood sugar (time/level): _____ / _____
_____ / _____
_____ / _____

EAT

Vegetables 0 1 2 3 4 5 6 7
Fruit 0 1 2 3
Smart protein 0 1 2 3
Smart carbs 0 1 2 3

Breakfast: _____ minutes
☐ Hungry ☐ Planned ☐ Portioned
Notes: _____

Lunch: _____ minutes
☐ Hungry ☐ Planned ☐ Portioned
Notes: _____

Dinner: _____ minutes
☐ Hungry ☐ Planned ☐ Portioned
Notes: _____

Snack: _____ minutes
☐ Hungry ☐ Planned ☐ Portioned
Notes: _____

MOVE

☐ Walked _____ minutes _____ steps
☐ Sugar Buster routine _____
☐ Found at least one opportunity to move

CHOOSE

Bedtime: _____
Wake time: _____
Bedtime routine: ☐
Self-care time: ☐ ☐ ☐ ☐ ☐
Deep breathing: ☐ ☐ ☐

My attitude:
☺ ☹ 😣 😰 ☺ 😁 😖

Week 6 Goals

EAT

NEW This week, you'll add smart fats to your Eat goals. Smarten up at least one of your daily fat servings by switching to olive or avocado oil, using smashed avocado in place of butter, snacking on nuts and seeds instead of chips, and choosing fatty fish such as salmon over fatty red meats. Make sure you watch your portion size when adding fats. You only need one tablespoon worth, which is the size of your thumb. See Goal 5 in the Eat chapter (page 63) for a refresher on smart fats.

Max out your veggie, protein, and fruit servings. Try to consume at least five veggie servings a day, three fruit servings a day, and protein with every main meal.

Smarten up at least two of your daily starch servings by opting for beans, lentils, potato (with the skin), whole grains, or another whole food instead of a highly processed option.

Continue to use the Reverse Diabetes plate for portion control. As a refresher, half of your plate is veggies, a quarter is protein, and a quarter is starch. Devote up to one tablespoon (the size of your thumb) for fat.

Make each meal last one or two minutes longer than the week before. Set a rule for yourself: You won't put more food in your mouth if food is still in your mouth.

Plan most of your dinners and some of your lunches.

Continue to wait until you feel stomach hungry before snacking as well as before meals.

MOVE

Move five minutes longer than you did last week. So if you walked 30 minutes most days, then your goal is 35 minutes most days this week.

Keep doing the Sugar Busters strength training routine this week. Do each sequence at least twice during the week.

Add more daily movement.

Smart Tip Have a goal.
Exercise is more fun when you're
working toward something specific.
Sign up for a charity walk, a 5K
run, or a golf tournament. Or keep
track of how much time you spend
exercising and treat yourself to a
massage when you reach, say,
500 minutes of exercise.

CHOOSE

Continue to improve on sleep and self-care.

Continue to breathe deeply before meals and
use your bedtime ritual.

NEW Develop a nourishment ritual. This is a
type of self-care you can turn to when you would
otherwise use food to cope. For example, instead
of inhaling a tub of ice cream when you're stressed,
take a long shower, go for a walk, or cuddle with
a pet. Consider what makes you feel loved, whole,
relaxed, and connected. Whenever you choose to
nourish your soul rather than mindlessly snacking, check the box on your habit tracker.

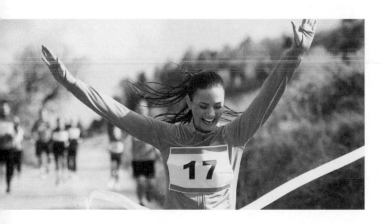

Habit Tracker

My numbers:

Weight or measurements: _____
Blood sugar (time/level): _____ / _____
_____ / _____
_____ / _____

EAT

Vegetables 0 1 2 3 4 5 6 7
Fruit 0 1 2 3
Smart protein 0 1 2 3
Smart carbs 0 1 2 3
Smart fats 0 1 2 3

Breakfast: _____ minutes
☐ Hungry ☐ Planned ☐ Portioned
Notes: _____

Lunch: _____ minutes
☐ Hungry ☐ Planned ☐ Portioned
Notes: _____

Dinner: _____ minutes
☐ Hungry ☐ Planned ☐ Portioned
Notes: _____

Snack: _____ minutes
☐ Hungry ☐ Planned ☐ Portioned
Notes: _____

MOVE

☐ Walked _____ minutes _____ steps
☐ Sugar Buster routine _____
☐ Found at least two opportunities to move

CHOOSE

Bedtime: _____
Wake time: _____
Bedtime routine: ☐
Self-care time: ☐ ☐ ☐ ☐ ☐
Deep breathing: ☐ ☐ ☐
Nourishment: ☐ ☐ ☐

My attitude:
☺ ☹ 😫 😣 ☺ 😁 😟

157

Week 7 Goals

EAT

Continue to swap out highly refined foods for smart carbs and smart fats. Try to consume at least five veggie servings a day, three fruit servings a day, and protein with every main meal. Choose smart carbs for most meals and snacks. Smarten up at least two of your daily fat servings.

Continue to use the Reverse Diabetes plate for portion control.

Continue to eat slowly. Set a rule for yourself: You will not put more food on your fork while a previous bite of food is still in your mouth.

Plan most of your dinners, most of your lunches, and some of your breakfasts and snacks.

Wait until you feel stomach hungry before eating most meals and snacks.

MOVE

Move five minutes longer than you did last week. So if you walked 35 minutes most days, then your goal is 40 minutes most days this week.

Keep doing the Sugar Busters strength training routine. Do each sequence at least twice during the week.

Keep adding daily movement. Consider signing up for a regular activity, such as pickleball, Zumba, or aqua yoga.

CHOOSE

Continue to improve on sleep and self-care, breathe deeply before meals, and use your nourishment rituals.

NEW Experiment with gratitude. During each day, search for ways to thank others around you. Aim for at least one thank you a day.

Smart Tip Leave peels on. Unpeeled fruits and vegetables contain more filling fiber than those with their skin and membranes removed. Wash or scrub unpeeled produce carefully with warm water. If you're concerned about pesticide residue, buy organic produce when you can afford it.

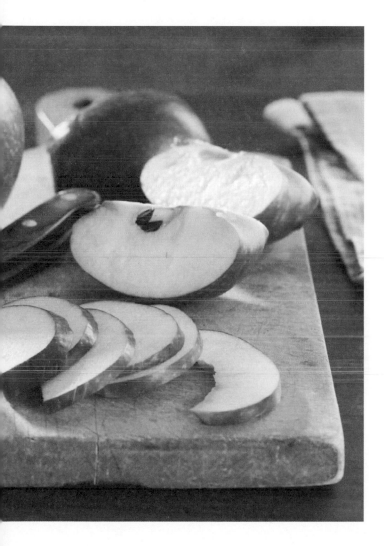

⑦ Habit Tracker

● **My numbers:**

Weight or measurements: _____

Blood sugar (time/level): _____/ _____
_____/ _____
_____/ _____

● **EAT**

Vegetables 0 1 2 3 4 5 6 7
Fruit 0 1 2 3
Smart protein 0 1 2 3
Smart carbs 0 1 2 3
Smart fats 0 1 2 3

Breakfast: _____ minutes
☐ Hungry ☐ Planned ☐ Portioned
Notes: _____

Lunch: _____ minutes
☐ Hungry ☐ Planned ☐ Portioned
Notes: _____

Dinner: _____ minutes
☐ Hungry ☐ Planned ☐ Portioned
Notes: _____

Snack: _____ minutes
☐ Hungry ☐ Planned ☐ Portioned
Notes: _____

● **MOVE**

☐ Walked _____ minutes _____ steps
☐ Sugar Buster routine _____
☐ Found at least two opportunities to move

● **CHOOSE**

Bedtime: _____
Wake time: _____
Bedtime routine: ☐
Self-care time: ☐ ☐ ☐ ☐ ☐
Deep breathing: ☐ ☐ ☐
Nourishment: ☐ ☐ ☐
Times I thanked people: ☐ ☐ ☐ ☐ ☐

● **My attitude:**
☺ ☹ 😣 😵 😐 😁 😖

Week 8 Goals

EAT

Continue to choose whole foods over refined foods. Consume at least five veggie servings a day, three fruit servings a day, and protein with every meal. Choose smart carbs and smart fats for most meals and snacks.

Use the Reverse Diabetes plate for portion control at most meals.

Eat slowly. Set a rule for yourself: You'll take a sip of water after every third bite of food.

Plan most of your dinners, most of your lunches, and most of your breakfasts and snacks.

Wait until you feel stomach hungry before eating most meals and snacks.

MOVE

Move five minutes longer than you did last week. So if you walked 40 minutes most days, then your goal is 45 minutes most days this week. That's your ultimate walking goal.

Keep doing the Sugar Busters strength training routine. Do each sequence at least twice during the week.

Keep adding daily movement. Look for ways to pair active time with podcasts, meetings, and other life activities.

CHOOSE

Continue to improve on sleep and self-care, breathe deeply before meals, use your nourishment rituals, and experiment with gratitude.

NEW Practice self-compassion. See page 136 in the Choose chapter for a refresher. Consider doing it at the end of the day, as part of your bedtime routine.

Smart Tip Eggs are a great source of protein so you don't need to shy away from eating them. But if you'd like to save some calories and saturated fat, replace a whole egg with two egg whites in recipes. Or use ground flaxseeds for a plant-based egg substitute. For each egg, add three tablespoons water to one tablespoon ground flaxseed and allow to stand for five minutes or until gelatinous.

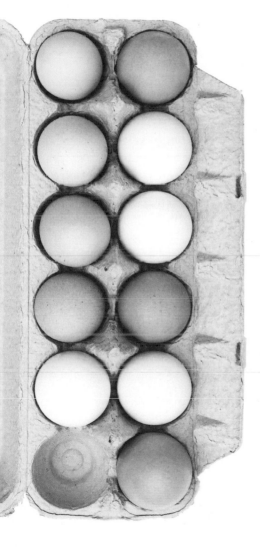

8 Habit Tracker

My numbers:

Weight or measurements: _____

Blood sugar (time/level): _____ / _____
_____ / _____
_____ / _____

EAT

Vegetables 0 1 2 3 4 5 6 7
Fruit 0 1 2 3
Smart protein 0 1 2 3
Smart carbs 0 1 2 3
Smart fats 0 1 2 3

Breakfast: _____ minutes
☐ Hungry ☐ Planned ☐ Portioned
Notes: _____

Lunch: _____ minutes
☐ Hungry ☐ Planned ☐ Portioned
Notes: _____

Dinner: _____ minutes
☐ Hungry ☐ Planned ☐ Portioned
Notes: _____

Snack: _____ minutes
☐ Hungry ☐ Planned ☐ Portioned
Notes: _____

MOVE

☐ Walked _____ minutes _____ steps
☐ Sugar Buster routine _____
☐ Found at least three opportunities to move

CHOOSE

Bedtime: _____
Wake time: _____
Bedtime routine: ☐
Self-care time: ☐ ☐ ☐ ☐ ☐
Deep breathing: ☐ ☐ ☐
Nourishment: ☐ ☐ ☐
Times I thanked people: ☐ ☐ ☐ ☐ ☐
Practiced self-compassion: ☐

My attitude:
☺ ☹ 😖 😷 🙂 😁 😫

Week 9 Goals

EAT

NEW Notice your stomach hunger before, during, and just after meals. Before digging in, rate your hunger on a scale of 0 (we couldn't pay you to eat right now) to 10 (you're so hungry you could eat this book). Do this again when you're about halfway through what's on your plate and again just after the last bite.

Continue to choose whole foods. Consume at least five veggie servings a day, three fruit servings a day, and protein with every meal. Choose smart carbs and smart fats for most meals and snacks.

Use the Reverse Diabetes plate for portion control.

Eat slowly. Experiment with ways to slow down, such as listening to slow-paced music, setting your flatware down between bites, or even looking at a note that says "slow down."

Plan most meals.

MOVE

NEW Now that you're walking 45 minutes or longer, it's time to add some faster segments. Warm up for 10 minutes with a slow stroll. Then set a timer to remind you to walk quickly—as if you are racing to catch a bus—for one minute out of every 10 for a total of three minutes of faster walking. Then cool down with slower walking.

Keep doing the Sugar Busters strength training routine. Do each sequence at least twice during the week.

Keep adding daily movement. Look for ways to pair active time with podcasts, meetings, and other life activities.

CHOOSE

Continue to improve on sleep and self-care, breathe deeply before meals, use your nourishment rituals, experiment with gratitude, and practice self-compassion.

NEW Look into ways you might give back to your community and meet your Move goals. Maybe you volunteer to walk dogs for a local animal shelter, for example.

Smart Tip Do you tend to eat when you're bored? If so, make a list of other things you can do in those instances, and post it on your refrigerator. Your list may include calling a friend, taking your dog for a walk, knitting, organizing your photos, or spending time on an old or new hobby.

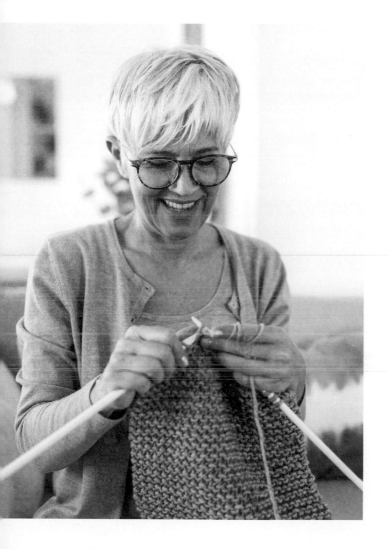

⑨ Habit Tracker

My numbers:

Weight or measurements: _____

Blood sugar (time/level): _____ / _____

_____ / _____

_____ / _____

EAT

Vegetables 0 1 2 3 4 5 6 7
Fruit 0 1 2 3
Smart protein 0 1 2 3
Smart carbs 0 1 2 3
Smart fats 0 1 2 3

Breakfast: _____ minutes
☐ Hungry ☐ Planned ☐ Portioned
Notes: _____

Lunch: _____ minutes
☐ Hungry ☐ Planned ☐ Portioned
Notes: _____

Dinner: _____ minutes
☐ Hungry ☐ Planned ☐ Portioned
Notes: _____

Snack: _____ minutes
☐ Hungry ☐ Planned ☐ Portioned
Notes: _____

MOVE

☐ Walked _____ min. ☐ ☐ ☐ Faster segments
☐ Sugar Buster routine _____
☐ Found at least three opportunities to move

CHOOSE

Bedtime: _____
Wake time: _____
Bedtime routine: ☐
Self-care time: ☐ ☐ ☐ ☐ ☐
Deep breathing: ☐ ☐ ☐
Nourishment: ☐ ☐ ☐
Times I thanked people: ☐ ☐ ☐ ☐ ☐
Practiced self-compassion: ☐

My attitude:
☺ ☹ 😖 😴 😐 😁 😣

Week 10 Goals

EAT

Continue to notice your stomach hunger before, during, and just after meals. Don't start eating until your hunger reaches a six out of 10. See if you can stop eating when your hunger drops below a four, even if you still have food on your plate.

Continue to consume whole foods. Eat at least five veggie servings a day, three fruit servings a day, and protein with every meal. Choose smart carbs and smart fats for most meals and snacks.

Use the Reverse Diabetes plate for portion control.

Eat slowly.

Plan most meals.

MOVE

Let's build on your faster walking segments. Warm up for 10 minutes with a slow stroll. Then walk quickly for two minutes out of every 10 for a total of six minutes of faster walking. Then cool down with slower walking.

Keep doing the Sugar Busters strength training routine. Do each sequence at least twice during the week.

Keep adding daily movement. Look for ways to pair active time with podcasts, meetings, and other life activities.

CHOOSE

Continue to improve on sleep and self-care, breathe deeply before meals, use your nourishment rituals, experiment with gratitude, and practice self-compassion.

NEW Notice how you talk to yourself. Would you say the same thing to a friend or a loved one? Try to speak to yourself with kindness.

Smart Tip Start dinner with soup or a big salad. Studies show that people who begin a meal with a clear soup (avoid cream-based soups) or green salad consume fewer calories overall at the meal. Plus, it's an easy way to add more vegetables to your diet. Just be mindful of salt content by choosing lower-sodium picks.

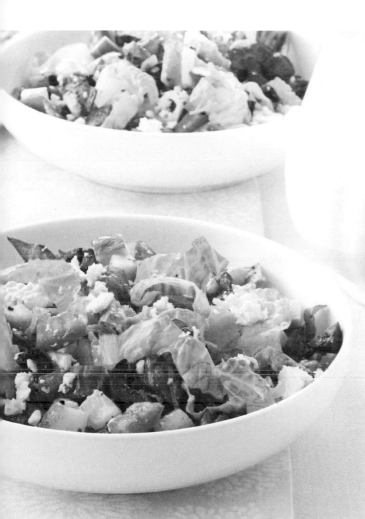

⑩ Habit Tracker

My numbers:

Weight or measurements: _____
Blood sugar (time/level): _____/ _____
_____/ _____
_____/ _____

EAT

Vegetables 0 1 2 3 4 5 6 7
Fruit 0 1 2 3
Smart protein 0 1 2 3
Smart carbs 0 1 2 3
Smart fats 0 1 2 3

Breakfast: _____ minutes
☐ Hungry ☐ Planned ☐ Portioned
Notes: _____

Lunch: _____ minutes
☐ Hungry ☐ Planned ☐ Portioned
Notes: _____

Dinner: _____ minutes
☐ Hungry ☐ Planned ☐ Portioned
Notes: _____

Snack: _____ minutes
☐ Hungry ☐ Planned ☐ Portioned
Notes: _____

MOVE

☐ Walked _____ min. ☐ ☐ ☐ Faster segments
☐ Sugar Buster routine _____
☐ Found at least three opportunities to move

CHOOSE

Bedtime: _____
Wake time: _____
Bedtime routine: ☐
Self-care time: ☐ ☐ ☐ ☐ ☐
Deep breathing: ☐ ☐ ☐
Nourishment: ☐ ☐ ☐
Times I thanked people: ☐ ☐ ☐ ☐ ☐
Practiced self-compassion: ☐

My attitude:
☺ ☹ 😖 😵 😐 😄 😣

Week 11 Goals

EAT

Shift your focus from building new habits to maintaining them. For the next two weeks, you won't find new tasks. Rather, you'll focus on taking what might feel like a struggle and turning it onto an automated habit.

Continue to notice your stomach hunger before, during, and just after meals. Try not to start eating until your hunger is at six. Try to stop eating when your hunger drops below four. If needed, reduce your portions by using an appetizer plate.

Continue to consume whole foods: Eat at least five veggie servings a day, three fruit servings a day, and protein with every meal as well as smart carbs and smart fats for most meals and snacks.

Use the Reverse Diabetes plate for portion control.

Eat slowly.

Plan most meals.

MOVE

Continue to build on your faster walking segments. Warm up for 10 minutes with a slow stroll. Then walk quickly for two minutes out of every eight. Then cool down with slower walking.

Keep doing the Sugar Busters strength training routine. Do each sequence at least twice during the week.

Maintain your daily movement. Look for ways to pair active time with podcasts, meetings, and other life activities.

CHOOSE

Maintain sleep and self-care, breathing deeply before meals, using your nourishment rituals, experimenting with gratitude, and practicing self-compassion.

Search for wins. Mentally give yourself a high five whenever you accomplish your Eat, Move, and Choose activities.

Smart Tip Discover fresh herbs. Add flavor to vegetables, salads, meat, poultry, and fish with fresh herbs such as basil, rosemary, parsley, oregano, and cilantro. Most grocery stores carry fresh herbs—or grow your own on a sunny windowsill.

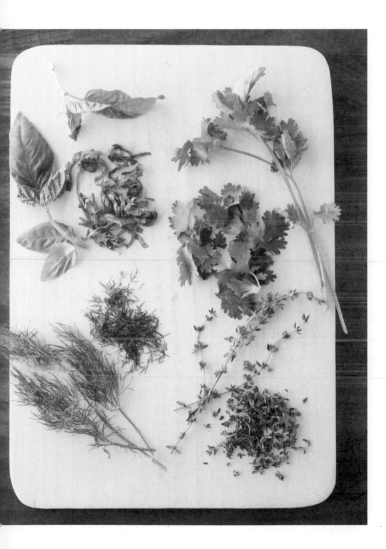

Habit Tracker

My numbers:

Weight or measurements: _____

Blood sugar (time/level): _____/ _____

_____/ _____

_____/ _____

EAT

Vegetables 0 1 2 3 4 5 6 7
Fruit 0 1 2 3
Smart protein 0 1 2 3
Smart carbs 0 1 2 3
Smart fats 0 1 2 3

Breakfast: _____ minutes
□ Hungry □ Planned □ Portioned
Notes: _____

Lunch: _____ minutes
□ Hungry □ Planned □ Portioned
Notes: _____

Dinner: _____ minutes
□ Hungry □ Planned □ Portioned
Notes: _____

Snack: _____ minutes
□ Hungry □ Planned □ Portioned
Notes: _____

MOVE

□ Walked _____ min. □ □ □ Faster segments
□ Sugar Buster routine _____
□ Found at least three opportunities to move

CHOOSE

Bedtime: _____
Wake time: _____
Bedtime routine: □
Self-care time: □ □ □ □ □
Deep breathing: □ □ □
Nourishment: □ □ □
Times I thanked people: □ □ □ □ □
Practiced self-compassion: □

My attitude:
☺ ☹ 😣 😴 ☺ 😁 😟

Week 12 Goals

EAT

Continue to notice your stomach hunger before, during, and just after meals. Don't start eating until your hunger reaches a six or seven. Stop eating once it dips below a four.

Continue to consume whole foods: Eat at least five veggie servings a day, three fruit servings a day, and protein with every meal as well as smart carbs and smart fats for most meals and snacks.

Use the Reverse Diabetes plate for portion control.

Eat slowly.

Plan most meals.

MOVE

Continue to build on your faster walking segments. Warm up for 10 minutes with a slow stroll. Walk quickly for two minutes, then recover by walking slowly for two minutes. Repeat for a total of 26 minutes combined. Then cool down with slower walking for 10 minutes.

Keep doing the Sugar Busters strength training routine. Do each sequence at least twice during the week.

Keep focusing on daily movement.

CHOOSE

Continue to maintain sleep and self-care, breathing deeply before meals, using your nourishment rituals and practicing gratitude and self-compassion.

NEW Schedule an appointment with your doctor to see how your health has improved during the past 12 weeks.

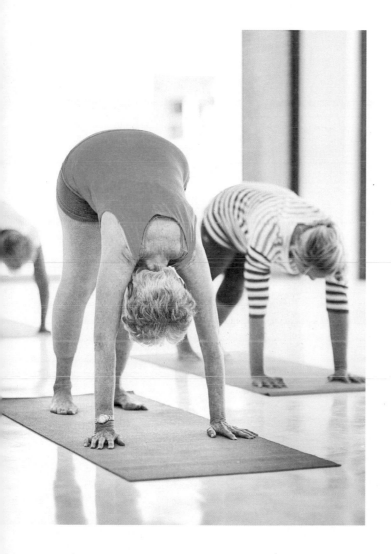

Smart Tip Exercise with a friend. Your walk, jog, or swim will be much more enjoyable—and probably longer—if you go with a companion. Also, a friend can be a great motivator: You're much less likely to skip a workout if you know your buddy is waiting for you.

12 Habit Tracker

My numbers:

Weight or measurements: _____

Blood sugar (time/level): _____ / _____

_____ / _____

_____ / _____

EAT

Vegetables 0 1 2 3 4 5 6 7
Fruit 0 1 2 3
Smart protein 0 1 2 3
Smart carbs 0 1 2 3
Smart fats 0 1 2 3

Breakfast: _____ minutes
☐ Hungry ☐ Planned ☐ Portioned
Notes: _____

Lunch: _____ minutes
☐ Hungry ☐ Planned ☐ Portioned
Notes: _____

Dinner: _____ minutes
☐ Hungry ☐ Planned ☐ Portioned
Notes: _____

Snack: _____ minutes
☐ Hungry ☐ Planned ☐ Portioned
Notes: _____

MOVE

☐ Walked _____ min. ☐ ☐ ☐ Faster segments
☐ Sugar Buster routine _____
☐ Found at least three opportunities to move

CHOOSE

Bedtime: _____
Wake time: _____
Bedtime routine: ☐
Self-care time: ☐ ☐ ☐ ☐
Deep breathing: ☐ ☐ ☐
Nourishment: ☐ ☐ ☐
Times I thanked people: ☐ ☐ ☐ ☐ ☐
Practiced self-compassion: ☐

My attitude:
☺ ☹ 😣 😓 😐 😁 😖

169

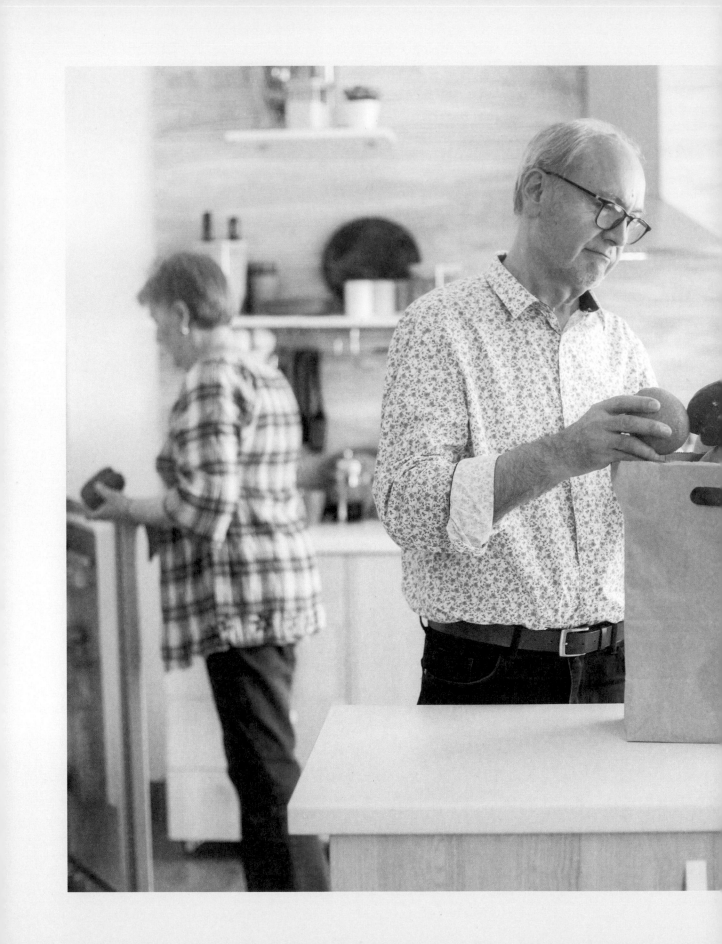

5

Reverse Diabetes
TOOLS

- Food Diary
- Organization Tools
- Shopping Help

Keep Yourself on Track to Better Health

IN THE FOLLOWING PAGES you'll find several tools that will make reversing diabetes *a lot* easier.

1. ***The Reverse Diabetes Kitchen Makeover*** will help set you up for success. Ideally, you'll want to do this before starting the 12-week challenge.

2. During your 12-week challenge, you'll want to turn to your Reverse Diabetes ***meal planner*** and ***shopping list*** over and over again. Each week write down what you plan to eat, then write out a corresponding shopping list of what groceries you'll need to make these meals. If you need inspiration for what to eat, check out the Reverse Diabetes Plate Ideas on pages 78-79 and the sample meal plans starting on page 241 for some ideas.

3. If you choose, keep a ***food diary*** during Week 1 to help you identify eating patterns you might want to change.

4. Next is ***a daily food and exercise log,*** which you can use if you'd like to more closely track the effects of specific foods and workouts on your blood sugar. (If you are already keeping a glucose log or tracking app, feel free to keep using that.)

5. If you find it easier to use than the blank shopping list template, we've included a ***grocery checklist*** that lists typical foods you'll need on the 12-week challenge so you can just check them off.

6. The remaining pages include a ***diabetes testing and management schedule*** and ***lists of calories, carbohydrates, fiber and glycemic loads for common foods*** for your reference.

These tools are all optional. We encourage you to check them out and decide for yourself whether they might ease your journey to a stronger, healthier you.

Exactly how you use these tools is up to you. You might photocopy them, use them as inspiration as you design your own tools, or download them from the Reverse Diabetes toolkit online at thehealthy.com/reversediabetes.

Scan to find the tools online.

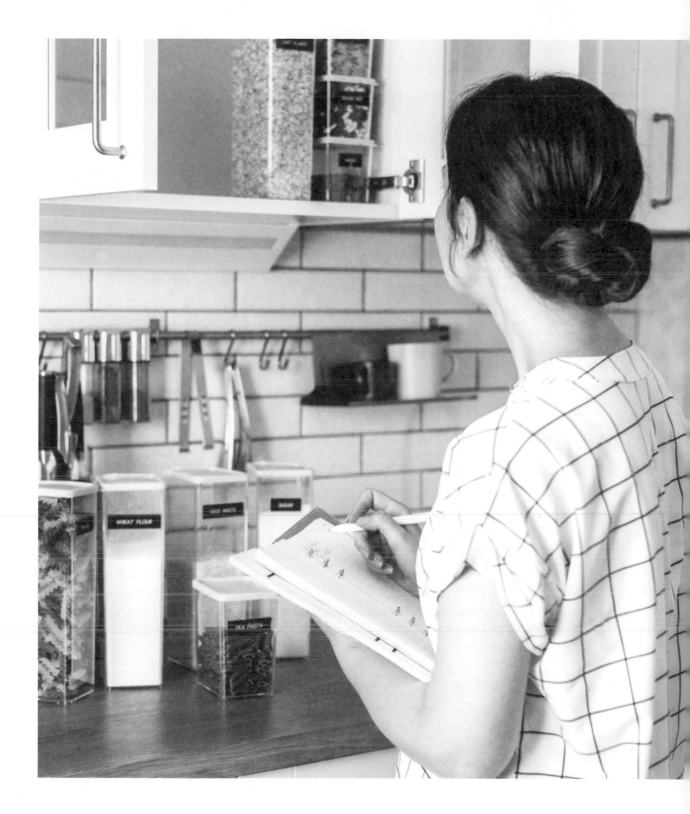

Reverse Diabetes Kitchen Makeover

A well-stocked, well-organized kitchen is your greatest Reverse Diabetes ally. Keeping the right foods at your fingertips means you'll be ready to put together fast, blood-sugar friendly meals and grab healthy treats when you want a snack. You'll be able to enjoy food without guilt, worry, fear—and without the danger of being sidetracked by temptations that make blood sugar spike and pack on pounds.

Ready to begin? The first step isn't shopping; it's clearing your kitchen of foods that pack too many calories or refined carbohydrates, too much saturated fat, or too much added sugar. Grab a bag for compostable food scraps and a box for items you can give away. (If there are items that other family members eat, put them in a designated area of the pantry, refrigerator, or freezer) The second step: Use our "Stock Up" list to put the right edibles in place.

No need to overspend the grocery budget; you can add a few to your shopping list each week. You can check them off here or go to thehealthy.com/reversediabetes/kitchenmakeover for a digital version of this list.

Scan to find the list online.

PANTRY

Give away, move to a designated spot, or compost:

- ☐ Boxed mashed potato mix
- ☐ Breakfast cereals high in added sugar or that don't list a whole grain as the first ingredient
- ☐ Butter-flavored microwave popcorn
- ☐ Candy
- ☐ Canned fruit in heavy syrup
- ☐ Cereal bars (except those that are low sugar, contain no hydrogenated oil, and list a whole grain as the first ingredient)
- ☐ Cookies
- ☐ Corn oil
- ☐ Crackers that contain hydrogenated oil or don't have a whole grain, seed, or vegetable as the first ingredient
- ☐ Cream soups
- ☐ Non-diet soda and juice drinks
- ☐ Packaged and snack foods that list hydrogenated oils or trans fats
- ☐ Sugar-sweetened iced tea or lemonade mix
- ☐ Shortening
- ☐ Chips
- ☐ White bread
- ☐ White rice

Stock

- ☐ Applesauce, no-sugar-added
- ☐ Broth—low-sodium chicken or vegetable
- ☐ Brown rice
- ☐ Cereal, whole-grain, with at least three grams of fiber per serving
- ☐ Cocoa powder, unsweetened
- ☐ Cooking spray
- ☐ Couscous, whole-grain
- ☐ Fruit, canned in juice or light syrup
- ☐ Garlic, fresh
- ☐ Legumes (black beans, chickpeas, etc.), canned or dried
- ☐ Mushrooms, dried
- ☐ Oils—olive, canola, avocado
- ☐ Onions
- ☐ Nut and seed butter
- ☐ Popcorn kernels
- ☐ Potatoes and sweet potatoes or yams
- ☐ Raisins, other dried fruit
- ☐ Salmon, canned
- ☐ Sugar substitute
- ☐ Soups—low-sodium broth-based soups, especially vegetable and bean soups
- ☐ Tomatoes, canned
- ☐ Tomato sauce, no salt added
- ☐ Tuna, canned in water
- ☐ Vegetables, canned
- ☐ Vinegars
- ☐ Whole grains—barley, oats (rolled and steel-cut, farro, bulgur, etc.)
- ☐ Whole-grain bread, mini bagels, and rolls
- ☐ Whole-grain crackers
- ☐ Whole-wheat flour
- ☐ Whole-grain pasta

REFRIGERATOR

Give away, move to a designated spot, or compost:

- [ ] Butter (or use very sparingly)
- [ ] Full-fat cheddar, jack, and other cheeses (or cut the cheese the recipe calls for in half)
- [ ] Full-fat milk, half-and-half, and cream
- [ ] Full-fat sour cream

- [ ] Full-fat yogurt
- [ ] Margarines that contain trans fats
- [ ] Sugary drinks—sodas, sweetened teas, fruit juice drinks

Stock

- [ ] Eggs and/or egg substitute
- [ ] Fruit, assorted fresh

- [ ] Hard cheese for grating, such as Parmesan
- [ ] Lean beef, chicken, turkey, or pork
- [ ] Margarine (with no trans fats and saturated fat)
- [ ] Milk—low-fat, nonfat or plant-based
- [ ] Nonfat or low-fat sour cream
- [ ] Nuts and seeds

- [ ] Plant-based meat alternatives
- [ ] Tempeh and/or tofu
- [ ] Vegetables, assorted fresh
- [ ] Yogurt, plain—low-fat or nonfat, sweetened with a no-calorie sweetener if desired

FREEZER

Give away, move to a designated spot, or compost:

- [ ] Bacon and full-fat breakfast sausage
- [ ] Breaded fish sticks, fish fillets, and chicken
- [ ] French fries and potato nuggets
- [ ] Frozen snack foods

- [ ] Frozen waffles (except whole-grain)
- [ ] Frozen dinners containing more than 15 grams of saturated fat per serving
- [ ] Full-fat ice cream
- [ ] Vegetables in butter or cream sauces

Stock

- [ ] Berries and other fruit, frozen without added sugar
- [ ] Breads—whole-wheat and whole-grain pita
- [ ] Chicken breasts, individually portioned
- [ ] Edamame

- [ ] Fish fillets (unbreaded), shelled shrimp, scallops
- [ ] Ground turkey or lean ground beef
- [ ] Meatless burgers
- [ ] Sugar-free frozen fruit pops or bars
- [ ] Vegetables, frozen without sauces

KITCHEN EQUIPMENT

- [ ] Two dishwasher-safe cutting boards (reserve one for vegetables and fruit, one for meat)
- [ ] Air fryer (if you have the space and budget)
- [ ] Aluminum foil
- [ ] Good-quality nonstick or cast-iron skillet (it

will allow you to sauté foods with very little oil)
- [ ] Freezer bags and containers
- [ ] Microwave-safe food storage containers
- [ ] Nonstick stir-fry pan
- [ ] Opaque storage containers for "treat"

foods for other family members (so you won't be tempted by the sight of the contents)
- [ ] Pot (with lid) large enough to cook soup, rice, or pasta
- [ ] Plastic wrap (or eco-friendly alternative)

- [ ] Salad spinner
- [ ] Sharp kitchen knives
- [ ] Silicone spatula
- [ ] Vegetable scrubber
- [ ] Vegetable steamer
- [ ] Zipper-lock bags

175

Meal Planner

List what you plan to eat for the week to come. Photocopy this to use from week to week or use the digital version at thehealthy.com/reversediabetes/mealplanner. You'll find a filled-in example of this planner on page 178.

Scan to find the planner online.

DAY	DINNER
Sunday	
Monday	
Tuesday	
Wednesday	
Thursday	
Friday	
Saturday	

BREAKFAST IDEAS

LUNCH IDEAS

SNACK IDEAS

Shopping List

As you plan meals, use this shopping list to jot down any ingredients you'll need at the store. Photocopy this to use from week to week or use the digital version at thehealthy.com/reversediabetes/shoppinglist. You'll find a filled-in example of this list on page 179.

PRODUCE

_____

_____

_____

_____

_____

_____

_____

_____

_____

_____

_____

MEAT AND POULTRY

_____

_____

_____

_____

FISH

_____

_____

_____

FROZEN FOODS

_____

_____

_____

_____

REFRIGERATED FOODS

_____

_____

_____

_____

_____

DELI

_____

_____

_____

PACKAGED GOODS

_____

_____

_____

_____

_____

_____

_____

SNACKS

_____

_____

_____

_____

_____

BEVERAGES

_____

_____

_____

_____

_____

OTHER

_____

_____

_____

_____

_____

Scan to find the list online.

Meal Planner Example

Here's an example of how you might plan your meals for the week and make a shopping list accordingly.

DAY	DINNER
Sunday	Homemade pizza night
Monday	Pulled chicken sandwiches with homemade slaw
Tuesday	Leftover pulled chicken and pasta
Wednesday	Burger night
Thursday	Breakfast for dinner
Friday	Eat out
Saturday	Roasted salmon with green beans

BREAKFAST IDEAS

Greek yogurt, sliced apple, and pumpkin seeds

Whole-wheat toast topped with mashed avocado and a fried egg

Two quinoa egg cups with fruit

LUNCH IDEAS

Big salad topped with roasted chicken and sliced avocado

Open-faced sandwich with leftover slaw and roast beef

Sweet potato "toast" topped with ricotta cheese and side salad with two hard-boiled eggs

SNACK IDEAS

Sliced apple with peanut butter

Blueberries topped with whipped cream

Celery sticks stuffed with hummus

Shopping List Example

PRODUCE

Mushrooms

Onions

Spinach

Shredded cabbage

Broccoli

Salad greens

Apples

Berries

Green beans

Avocado

Sweet potato

Celery

_____

MEAT AND POULTRY

Chicken thighs

Turkey bacon

Ground turkey

Rotisserie chicken

_____

FISH

Salmon

_____

_____

FROZEN FOODS

_____

_____

_____

_____

_____

REFRIGERATED FOODS

Shredded cheese

Eggs

Greek yogurt

Ricotta

Whipped cream

Prepared hummus

_____

DELI

Deli roast beef

_____

_____

_____

_____

_____

_____

PACKAGED GOODS

Yeast

Whole-grain flour

Tomato sauce

BBQ sauce

Lentil pasta

Protein pancake mix

Pumpkin seeds

Quinoa

Peanut butter

_____

_____

SNACKS

_____

_____

_____

_____

_____

_____

_____

BEVERAGES

_____

_____

_____

_____

_____

_____

_____

OTHER

Whole-grain
  burger buns

Whole-grain bread

_____

_____

_____

_____

179

Your Food Diary

If you would like to get a better understanding of your eating patterns, in Week 1 of your Reverse Diabetes challenge, fill out this food diary after each meal or snack. Photocopy this to use from day to day or use the digital version at thehealthy.com/reversediabetes/fooddiary. You'll find two filled-in examples of this diary on the next page. At the end of the week, look over your diary for patterns and opportunities. Do you never eat a fruit or vegetable at breakfast or lunch? Do you snack late at night? Where are you overdoing the calories?

Scan to find the diary online.

DATE	TIME	WHAT I ATE/DRANK	NOTES
Breakfast			
Lunch			
Dinner			
Snacks			

Your Food Diary Example

DATE May 23	TIME	WHAT I ATE/DRANK	NOTES
Breakfast	7 a.m.	3 scrambled eggs; 2 slices toast; 1 Tbsp. butter; 6 oz. orange juice	Feeling rushed
Lunch	1:30 p.m.	Sandwich: 3 oz. turkey, 3 oz. cheese, 2 slices bread, ½ tsp. mayo; apple; 8 oz. potato chips; 1 12-oz. cola	Ate at desk; really hungry
Dinner	7:30 p.m.	3 BBQ chicken thighs; 1 corn on cob; 1 cup watermelon chunks; 1 12-oz. beer	
Snacks	4 p.m.	Cake; 2 Tbsp. mixed nuts	Office party

DATE June 15	TIME	WHAT I ATE/DRANK	NOTES
Breakfast	7 a.m.	1 jar overnight oats: ½ cup oats, ½ cup milk, ¼ cup Greek yogurt, 1 Tbsp. chia, 1 Tbsp. syrup, ¼ cup berries	Remembered to prep!
Lunch	12:30 p.m.	Rice bowl: 6 oz. grilled chicken, 1 cup brown rice, handful carrot/cabbage slaw, ½ cup cubed roasted sweet potatoes, 1 Tbsp. ginger miso dressing	Assembled night before!
Dinner	7 p.m.	6 oz. roasted salmon; ½ baked potato; 1 cup roasted broccoli	
Snacks	3:30 p.m.	1 popsicle; veggies with 1 Tbsp. hummus	

Daily Food and Exercise Log

If you choose, you can use this log to more closely track the effects of specific foods and workouts on your blood sugar. Photocopy this to use from day to day or find a digital version at thehealthy.com/reversediabetes/foodexerciselog.

Scan to find the log online.

Day:_____ Date:_____

MORNING

Breakfast Time:_____ Blood sugar before eating:_____

ITEM	AMOUNT	CARBS*

Blood sugar two hours after eating:_____

Snack Time:_____ Blood sugar before eating:_____

ITEM	AMOUNT	CARBS*

Exercise Time:_____

ACTIVITY
_____
_____
_____
_____
_____

DURATION
_____
_____

MIDDAY

Lunch Time:_____ Blood sugar before eating:_____

ITEM	AMOUNT	CARBS*

Blood sugar two hours after eating:_____

Snack Time:_____ Blood sugar before eating:_____

ITEM	AMOUNT	CARBS*

Exercise Time:_____

ACTIVITY
_____
_____
_____
_____
_____

DURATION
_____
_____

EVENING

Dinner Time:_____ Blood sugar before eating:_____

ITEM	AMOUNT	CARBS*

Blood sugar two hours after eating:_____

Snack Time:_____ Blood sugar before eating:_____

ITEM	AMOUNT	CARBS*

Exercise Time:_____

ACTIVITY
_____
_____
_____
_____
_____

DURATION
_____
_____

*choices or grams

Grocery Checklist

If you prefer, you can make a dozen copies of this list and post one each week on your refrigerator. Use the check-off boxes to note what you need so that grocery shopping's a breeze. Or use the digital version at thehealthy.com/reversediabetes/grocerychecklist.

FRUITS

- ☐ Apples
- ☐ Bananas
- ☐ Berries
- ☐ Grapes
- ☐ Kiwifruit
- ☐ Lemons/limes
- ☐ Mangoes
- ☐ Melons
- ☐ Oranges
- ☐ Peaches/nectarines/ apricots
- ☐ Pears
- ☐ Plums
- ☐ Other:

_____

_____

_____

VEGETABLES

- ☐ Asparagus
- ☐ Bell peppers
- ☐ Broccoli
- ☐ Carrots
- ☐ Cauliflower
- ☐ Celery
- ☐ Corn
- ☐ Cucumbers
- ☐ Eggplant
- ☐ Garlic
- ☐ Green beans
- ☐ Kale, collards, and other greens for cooking
- ☐ Mushrooms
- ☐ Onions
- ☐ Potatoes (sweet and white)
- ☐ Salad greens
- ☐ Spinach
- ☐ Tomatoes
- ☐ Winter squash
- ☐ Zucchini/summer squash
- ☐ Other:

_____

_____

_____

MEAT AND SEAFOOD

- ☐ Chicken or turkey breast
- ☐ Lean beef (round, sirloin, flank steak, tenderloin)
- ☐ Lean pork (ham, tenderloin, center loin chop)
- ☐ Fresh fish or seafood
- ☐ Other:

_____

_____

REFRIGERATOR CASE

- ☐ Eggs
- ☐ Low-fat cheeses
- ☐ Tofu
- ☐ Low-fat yogurt
- ☐ Margarine
- ☐ Milk (nonfat, low-fat, or plant-based)

GRAINS

- ☐ Barley
- ☐ Bulgur
- ☐ Oats, rolled and steel-cut
- ☐ Rice, brown or converted
- ☐ Whole grain (farro, freekeh, quinoa, etc.)
- ☐ Whole-grain cereal
- ☐ Whole-grain bread
- ☐ Whole-grain crackers
- ☐ Whole-grain pasta
- ☐ Other:

_____

_____

_____

NONPERISHABLES

- ☐ Cooking spray
- ☐ Gelatin
- ☐ Nuts (almonds, walnuts, peanuts)
- ☐ Oils (avocado, olive, canola)
- ☐ Peanut butter and other nut butters
- ☐ Stevia or other sugar substitutes

CANNED GOODS

- ☐ Beans (black, kidney, navy, etc.)
- ☐ Soup (low-sodium, bean/vegetable)
- ☐ Tomatoes
- ☐ Other vegetables (artichoke hearts, roasted peppers)
- ☐ Tuna packed in water
- ☐ Canned fruit in juice or light syrup

FREEZER AISLE

- ☐ Frozen fish fillets (without breading or sauce)
- ☐ Frozen shrimp and/or scallops
- ☐ Frozen vegetables
- ☐ Frozen fruit (without added sugar)
- ☐ Veggie burgers
- ☐ Sugar-free frozen fruit pops or bars
- ☐ Other:

_____

_____

_____

OTHER

_____

_____

_____

_____

Scan to find the list online.

Diabetes Testing and Management Schedule

Scan to find the schedule online.

At Every Doctor's Visit (usually four times per year)

TEST	DATE	RESULT	DATE	RESULT	DATE	RESULT	DATE	RESULT
A1C (goal is lower than 7)								
Blood pressure (goal is lower than 130/80)								
Foot check								

Twice a Year

TEST	DATE	DATE
Dental cleaning and exam		

Yearly (on anniversary of last test)

TEST	LAST YEAR'S DATE	LAST YEAR'S RESULT	THIS YEAR'S DATE	THIS YEAR'S RESULT
Microalbumin urine test (for kidney function)				
Eye exam (with dilation)				
LDL cholesterol*				
HDL cholesterol**				
Triglycerides***				
Foot exam (from a podiatrist)				
Flu shot				

*goal is lower than 100 mg/dl or lower than 70 mg/dl if you have known cardiovascular disease

**goal is higher than 40 mg/dl for men and higher than 50 mg/dl for women

***goal is lower than 150 mg/dl

Handy Numbers to Know

GENERAL BLOOD SUGAR TARGETS

Fasting or before-meal glucose	90–130 mg/dl
After-meal glucose (two hours after the start of your meal)	>180 mg/dl
Bedtime glucose	100–140 mg/dl

HOW TO TRANSLATE A1C NUMBERS

A1C	Blood Glucose Level	
6.0%	135 mg/dl	7.5 mmol/l*
6.5%	153 mg/dl	8.5 mmol/l*
7.0%	170 mg/dl	9.5 mmol/l*
7.5%	188 mg/dl	10.5 mmol/l*
8.0%	205 mg/dl	11.4 mmol/l*
8.5%	223 mg/dl	12.4 mmol/l*
9.0%	240 mg/dl	13.3 mmol/l*
9.5%	258 mg/dl	14.3 mmol/l*
10.0%	275 mg/dl	15.3 mmol/l*
10.5%	293 mg/dl	16.3 mmol/l*
11.0%	310 mg/dl	17.2 mmol/l*
11.5%	328 mg/dl	18.2 mmol/l*
12.0%	345 mg/dl	19.1 mmol/l*

* Millimoles per liter, used outside the U.S.

HEALTHY WAIST CIRCUMFERENCE

Men	up to 40 inches
Women	up to 35 inches

If your waist is bigger than this, you are at increased risk for type 2 diabetes, high blood pressure, high cholesterol, and cardiovascular disease.

Calories, Carbohydrates, and Fiber in Common Foods

Item	Amount	Calories	Carb grams	Fiber grams
BEEF				
Beef, chuck	3 oz.	293	0	0
Corned beef	3 oz.	213	0.8	0
Ground beef, 75% lean	3 oz.	236	0	0
Ground beef, 85% lean	3 oz.	213	0	0
Beef, rib	3 oz.	304	0	0
Beef, bottom round	3 oz.	210	0	0
Beef, top sirloin	3 oz.	207	0	0
BEVERAGES				
Beer, light	12 fl oz.	103	5.2	0
Beer, regular	12 fl oz.	138	10.7	0
Chocolate milk	1 cup	226	31.7	1.1
Club soda	12 fl oz.	0	0	0
Coffee	6 fl oz.	2	0	0
Cola	12 fl oz.	155	39.8	0
Diet cola	12 fl oz.	4	0.4	0
Espresso	2 fl oz.	1	0	0
Fruit punch	8 fl oz.	117	29.7	0.5
Hot cocoa	1 cup	113	24	1
Ginger ale	12 fl oz.	124	32.1	0
Instant coffee	6 fl oz.	4	0.6	0
Lemonade	8 fl oz.	112	34.1	0.2
Liquor (rum, gin, vodka, whiskey)	1.5 fl oz.	110	0	0
Piña colada	4.5 fl oz.	245	32	0.4
Soy milk	1 cup	127	12.08	3.2
Tea	6 fl oz.	2	0.5	0
Wine, red	3.5 fl oz.	74	1.8	0
Wine, white	3.5 fl oz.	70	0.8	0
BREAD, BAGELS, ROLLS				
Bagel, plain	4"	245	48	2
Bagel, cinnamon raisin	4"	244	49	2
Bagel, egg	4"	247	47.2	2
Biscuit, buttermilk	4"	358	45.1	1.5
Bread, French	½" slice	69	13	0.8

Item	Amount	Calories	Carb grams	Fiber grams
Bread, Italian	1 slice	54	10	0.5
Bread, white	1 slice	67	12.7	0.6
Bread, wheat	1 slice	69	12.9	1.9
Bread, rye	1 slice	83	15.5	1.9
Bread, pumpernickel	1 slice	80	15.2	2.1
Bread, raisin	1 slice	71	13.6	1.1
Croissant	1	231	26.1	1.5
Corn bread	1 piece	173	28.3	1.4
Pita	4"	77	15.6	0.6
CEREALS				
All Bran	½ cup	79	23	9.7
Apple Cinnamon Cheerios	¾ cup	118	25	1.6
Cap'n Crunch	¾ cup	108	22.9	0.7
Cheerios	1 cup	111	22.2	3.6
Chex, Corn	1 cup	112	25.8	0.6
Chex, Honey Nut	¾ cup	117	26	0.4
Chex, Multi-Bran	1 cup	165	41	6.4
Cornflakes	1 cup	101	24.4	0.7
Cream of Wheat	1 cup	126	26.9	1
Froot Loops	1 cup	118	26.2	0.8
Frosted Flakes	¾ cup	114	28	1
Frosted Mini-Wheats	1 cup	173	42	5.5
Honey Nut Cheerios	1 cup	115	24	1.6
Life	¾ cup	121	25	2
Oatmeal, regular	1 cup	147	25.3	4
Oatmeal, instant, apples and cinnamon	1 packet	130	26.5	2.7
Puffed Rice	1 cup	56	12.6	0.2
Puffed Wheat	1 cup	44	10	0.5
Raisin Bran	1 cup	195	46.5	7.3
Rice Krispies	1 1/4 cups	119	28	0.1
Special K	1 cup	117	22	0.7
Shredded Wheat	2 biscuits	155	36.2	5.5
Total	¾ cup	105	24	2.6

Item	Amount	Calories	Carb grams	Fiber grams
Trix	1 cup	122	26	0.7
Wheaties	1 cup	107	26.7	3

DAIRY AND EGGS

Item	Amount	Calories	Carb grams	Fiber grams
Butter	1 Tbsp.	102	0	0
Cheese food, American	1 oz.	94	2.2	0
Cheese spread	1 oz.	82	2.5	0
Cheese, blue	1 oz.	100	0.7	0
Cheese, cheddar	1 oz.	114	0.4	0
Cheese, cottage, regular	1 cup	216	5.6	0
Cheese, cottage, 2% milk fat	1 cup	203	8.2	0
Cheese, cottage, 1% milk fat	1 cup	163	6.2	0
Cheese, cream	1 Tbsp.	51	0.4	0
Cheese, feta	1 oz.	75	1.2	0
Cheese, mozzarella, part skim milk	1 oz.	72	0.79	0
Cheese, mozzarella, whole milk	1 oz.	85	0.6	0
Cheese, Muenster	1 oz.	104	0.3	0
Cheese, Parmesan	1 Tbsp.	22	0.2	0
Cheese, American	1 oz.	106	0.5	0
Cheese, provolone	1 oz.	100	0.6	0
Cheese, ricotta, part skim milk	1 cup	339	12.6	0
Cheese, ricotta, whole milk	1 cup	428	7.5	0
Cheese, Swiss	1 oz.	108	1.5	0
Cream, half and half	1 Tbsp.	20	0.7	0
Cream, heavy whipping	1 Tbsp.	52	0.4	0
Cream, light	1 Tbsp.	29	0.6	0
Cream, sour	1 Tbsp.	26	0.5	0
Cream, sour, reduced-fat	1 Tbsp.	20	0.6	0
Cream, sour, fat-free	1 Tbsp.	12	2	0
Egg, whole	large	74	0.8	0
Egg, white	large	17	0.2	0
Egg, yolk	large	53	0.6	0
Eggnog	1 cup	343	34.3	0
Ice cream, chocolate	½ cup	143	18.6	0.8

Item	Amount	Calories	Carb grams	Fiber grams
Ice cream, vanilla, soft-serve	½ cup	191	19.1	0.6
Ice cream, vanilla	½ cup	133	15.6	0.5
Milkshake, vanilla	11 fl oz.	351	55.6	0
Buttermilk	1 cup	98	11.7	0
Milk, condensed, sweetened	1 cup	982	166.5	0
Milk, evaporated, nonfat	1 cup	200	29.1	0
Milk, nonfat	1 cup	83	12.1	0
Milk, 1% milk fat	1 cup	102	12.2	0
Milk, 2% milk fat	1 cup	102	11.4	0
Milk, whole	1 cup	146	11	0
Yogurt, fruit, low-fat	8 oz.	232	43.2	0
Yogurt, plain, low-fat	8 oz.	143	16	0

FATS AND OIL

Item	Amount	Calories	Carb grams	Fiber grams
Lard	1 Tbsp.	115	0	0
Margarine	1 Tbsp.	102	0.1	0
Margarine-like spread	1 Tbsp.	51	0	0
Mayonnaise, regular	1 Tbsp.	99	0	0
Mayonnaise, fat-free	1 Tbsp.	12	2	0.6
Oil, canola	1 Tbsp.	124	0	0
Oil, olive	1 Tbsp.	119	0	0
Oil, peanut	1 Tbsp.	119	0	0
Oil, sesame	1 Tbsp.	120	0	0
Oil, vegetable or corn	1 Tbsp.	120	0	0
Shortening	1 Tbsp.	113	0	0

FISH AND SHELLFISH

Item	Amount	Calories	Carb grams	Fiber grams
Catfish, breaded and fried	3 oz.	195	6.8	0.6
Crab	3 oz.	82	0	0
Flounder	3 oz.	99	0	0
Haddock, baked	3 oz.	95	0	0
Halibut	3 oz.	119	0	0
Lobster	3 oz.	83	1.1	0
Ocean perch	3 oz.	103	0	0
Orange roughy	3 oz.	76	0	0
Pollock	3 oz.	96	0	0

continued >>>

Item	Amount	Calories	Carb grams	Fiber grams
Rainbow trout	3 oz.	144	0	0
Raw clams	3 oz.	63	2.2	0
Raw oysters	6 med.	57	3.3	0
Salmon, baked or broiled	3 oz.	184	0	0
Salmon, canned	3 oz.	118	0	0
Sardines	3 oz.	177	0	0
Scallops, breaded	6 large	200	9.4	0
Shrimp, breaded	3 oz.	206	5.2	0.2
Swordfish	3 oz.	132	0	0
Tuna, baked or broiled	3 oz.	118	0	0
Tuna, chunk white	3 oz.	109	0	0

FRUIT AND JUICES

Item	Amount	Calories	Carb grams	Fiber grams
Apple juice	1 cup	117	29	0.2
Apple	1	72	19.1	3.3
Applesauce, sweetened	1 cup	194	51	3.1
Applesauce, unsweetened	1 cup	108	28	2.9
Apricot	1	17	3.9	0.7
Apricots, dried	¼ cup	96	25	3.6
Apricots, canned in heavy syrup	1 cup	214	55	4.1
Apricots, canned in juice	1 cup	117	30	3.9
Apricot nectar, canned	1 cup	141	36	1.5
Asian pear	1 small	51	13	4.4
Avocado	1 oz.	47	2.5	1.9
Banana	1	105	27	3.1
Blackberries	1 cup	75	18	7.6
Blueberries	1 cup	83	21	3.5
Cantaloupe	1 cup	107	28	3
Cherries, sour	1 cup	88	22	2.7
Cherries, sweet	10	49	11	1.6
Cranberries, dried, sweetened	¼ cup	92	24	2.5
Cranberry juice cocktail	8 fl oz.	144	36.4	0.3
Cranberry sauce, canned	1 slice	86	22	0.6
Currants, dried	¼ cup	102	26.7	2.4
Dates, chopped	¼ cup	122	32.7	3.3
Figs, dried	¼ cup	127	32.5	5.8

Item	Amount	Calories	Carb grams	Fiber grams
Figs, fresh	1	37	9.6	1.7
Grape juice	1 cup	154	37.9	0.3
Grapefruit	½	39	9.9	1.3
Grapefruit juice	1 cup	96	22.7	0.2
Grapes, red or green	1 cup	110	29	1.4
Kiwi	1	46	11.1	2.3
Honeydew melon	1 cup	60	16	1
Lemon juice	juice of 1 lemon	12	4	0.2
Lime juice	juice of 1 lime	10	3.2	0.2
Mandarin oranges, canned in light syrup	1 cup	154	41	1.8
Mango	1 cup	107	28	3.7
Nectarine	1	67	16.0	2.2
Orange juice	1 cup	112	25.8	0.5
Orange	1	62	15.4	3.1
Papaya	1 cup	55	29.8	2.5
Peach	1	38	9.4	1.5
Peaches, canned in heavy syrup	1 cup	194	52	3.4
Peaches, canned in juice	1 cup	109	29	3.2
Pear	1 pear	96	25.7	5.1
Pears, canned in heavy syrup	1 cup	197	51	4.3
Pears, canned in juice	1 cup	124	32	4
Pineapple juice	1 cup	140	34.5	0.5
Pineapple	1 cup	74	19.6	2.2
Pineapple, canned in heavy syrup	1 cup	198	51	2
Pineapple, canned in juice	1 cup	149	39	2
Plantain, raw	1	218	57	4.1
Plantain, cooked slices	1 cup	179	48	3.5
Plum	1	30	7.5	0.9
Plums, canned in heavy syrup	1 cup	230	60	2.6
Plums, canned in juice	1 cup	146	38	2.5
Prunes, dried	5	100	26	3

Item	Amount	Calories	Carb grams	Fiber grams
Prunes, stewed	1 cup	265	70	16.4
Prune juice	1 cup	182	44.7	2.6
Raisins	¼ cup	108	28.7	1.3
Raspberries	1 cup	64	14.7	8
Strawberries	1 cup	53	12.8	3.3
Tangerine	1	31	7.8	1.6
Watermelon	1 cup	56	11.5	0.6

GRAINS AND PASTAS

Item	Amount	Calories	Carb grams	Fiber grams
Couscous	1 cup	176	36.5	2.2
Barley, pearled and cooked	1 cup	193	44	6
Bulgur	1 cup	151	33	8.2
Cornmeal	1 cup	444	94	8.9
Egg noodles	1 cup	213	39.7	1.8
Kasha (buckwheat groats)	1 cup	155	33	4.5
Oat bran (raw)	1 cup	231	62.3	14.5
Rice, brown	1 cup	216	45	3.5
Rice, white	1 cup	205	45	0.6
Rice, instant	1 cup	162	35	1
Rice, wild	1 cup	166	35	3
Pasta, regular	1 cup	197	40	2.4
Pasta, whole-wheat	1 cup	174	37	6.3
Wheat flour, bleached (white)	1 cup	455	95	3.4
Wheat flour, whole grain	1 cup	407	87	14.6
Wheat germ	1 Tbsp.	27	3	0.9

LAMB, VEAL, AND GAME

Item	Amount	Calories	Carb grams	Fiber grams
Lamb, leg	3 oz.	219	0	0
Lamb, loin	3 oz.	265	0	0
Lamb, shoulder	3 oz.	294	0	0
Veal, leg	3 oz.	179	0	0
Duck	½ duck	144	0	0

LEGUMES

Item	Amount	Calories	Carb grams	Fiber grams
Baked beans	1 cup	239	53.9	10.4
Black beans	1 cup	227	40.8	15
Chickpeas	1 cup	185	32.7	7.9
Great northern beans	1 cup	209	37.3	12.4
Lentils	1 cup	230	39.9	15.6
Navy beans	1 cup	255	47.4	19.1
Pinto beans	1 cup	245	44.8	15.4
Red kidney beans	1 cup	225	40.4	13.1

NUTS AND SEEDS

Item	Amount	Calories	Carb grams	Fiber grams
Almonds	1 oz.	164	5.6	3.3
Brazil nuts	1 oz.	186	3.5	2.1
Cashews	1 oz.	163	9.3	1
Chestnuts	1 cup	350	75.7	7.3
Hazelnuts	1 oz.	178	4.7	2.7
Macadamia nuts	1 oz.	203	3.6	2.3
Peanuts	1 oz.	166	6.1	2.3
Pecans	1 oz.	196	3.9	2.7
Pistachios	1 oz.	161	7.6	2.9
Pumpkin seeds	1 oz.	148	3.8	1.1
Sesame seeds	1 Tbsp.	47	1.2	1
Sunflower seeds	1 oz.	165	6.8	2.9
Walnuts	1 oz.	185	3.9	1.9

PORK

Item	Amount	Calories	Carb grams	Fiber grams
Pork sausage	1 patty	92	0	0
Bacon	3 med. slices	103	0.3	0
Ham, roasted	3 oz.	207	0	0
Pork, loin chops	3 oz.	235	0	0
Pork, roast	3 oz.	217	0	0
Pork, shoulder	3 oz.	280	0	0
Pork, spareribs	3 oz.	337	0	0

continued >>>

Item	Amount	Calories	Carb grams	Fiber grams
POULTRY				
Chicken roll	2 slices	87	1.4	0
Chicken, breast w/o skin	½ breast	142	0	0
Chicken, dark meat w/o skin	1 drumstick	76	0	0
Chicken, thigh w/o skin	1 thigh	109	0	0
Chicken, breast w/ skin, batter-fried	½ breast	364	12.6	0.4
Chicken, dark meat w/ skin, batter-fried	1 drumstick	193	6	0.2
Chicken, thigh w/ skin, batter-fried	1 thigh	238	7.8	0.3
Turkey, roasted, dark	3 oz.	157	0	0
Turkey, roasted, light	3 oz.	132	0	0
SAUSAGE AND LUNCH MEAT				
Bologna	2 slices	175	3.1	0
Chicken, white meat	2 slices	72	1.3	0
Chicken breast, roasted, fat free	2 slices	48	0.9	0
Cooked salami	2 slices	142	1.3	0
Ham, regular	2 slices	91	2.1	0.7
Ham, extra lean	2 slices	60	0.4	0
Hard salami	2 slices	77	0.8	0
Sausage, pork or beef	2 links	103	0.7	0
Turkey breast	2 slices	55	1.8	0
Turkey breast, fat free	2 slices	47	2.52	0
Vienna sausage	1	37	0.4	0
SNACKS				
Chex Mix	1 oz.	120	8.5	1.6
Cheese puffs	1 oz.	157	15.3	0.3
Crackers, saltine	4	51	8.5	0.4

Item	Amount	Calories	Carb grams	Fiber grams
Granola bar, plain	1 bar	134	18.3	1.5
Olives	5 large	25	1.4	0.7
Pickles, dill	1	12	2.7	0.8
Popcorn, air-popped	1 cup	31	6.2	1.2
Popcorn, oil-popped	1 cup	55	6	1.1
Potato chips	1 oz.	155	14.5	1
Pretzels	10	229	47.5	1.9
Rice cakes	1 cake	35	7.3	0.4
Tortilla chips	1 oz.	142	17.8	1.8
SOUPS, GRAVIES, AND SAUCES				
Barbecue sauce	1 Tbsp.	12	2	0.2
Beef bouillon	1 cup	29	1.8	0
Beef gravy	¼ cup	31	2.8	0.2
Cheese sauce	¼ cup	110	4.3	0.3
Chicken gravy	¼ cup	47	3.2	0.2
Chicken noodle soup	1 cup	75	9.4	0.7
Country sausage gravy	¼ cup	96	3.9	0.4
Cream of mushroom soup	1 cup	129	9.3	0.5
Hot pepper sauce	1 tsp.	1	0.1	0
Lentil soup	1 cup	126	20.3	5
Manhattan clam chowder	1 cup	78	12.2	1.5
Minestrone	1 cup	82	11.2	1
Mushroom gravy	¼ cup	30	3.3	0.2
New England clam chowder	1 cup	164	16.7	1.5
Onion soup	1 cup	27	5.1	1
Pasta sauce	1 cup	185	28.2	1
Pea soup	1 cup	165	26.5	2.8
Salsa	1 Tbsp.	4	1	0.3
Teriyaki sauce	1 Tbsp.	15	2.9	0
Tomato soup	1 cup	85	16.6	0.5
Turkey gravy	¼ cup	30	3	0.2
Vegetable beef soup	1 cup	78	10.2	0.5

Item	Amount	Calories	Carb grams	Fiber grams
SWEETS				
Brownies	1	227	35.8	1.2
Chocolate chip cookies	1 cookie	49	9.3	0.4
Cinnamon roll	1 roll	223	30.5	1.4
Cake, pound	1 piece	109	13.7	0.1
Cake, chocolate w/o frosting	1 piece	340	50.7	1.5
Coffee cake, crumb-type	1 piece	263	29	1.3
Doughnut, plain	1	198	23.4	0.7
Doughnut, glazed	1	242	26.6	0.7
Fudge	1 piece	70	13	0.3
Graham crackers	2	59	10.8	0.2
Hard candy	1 small piece	12	2.9	0
Jellybeans	10 large	106	26.5	0.1
Marshmallows	1 cup	159	40.7	0.1
Milk chocolate	1 bar	235	26.2	1.5
Pie, apple	1 piece	411	57.5	1.9
Pie, pecan	1 piece	503	63.7	4
Pie, pumpkin	1 piece	316	40.9	2.9
Pineapple upside down cake	1 piece	267	58	0.9
Pudding, chocolate	½ cup	154	27.8	0.6
Semisweet chocolate pieces	1 cup	805	106.1	9.9
Snickers	1 bar	266	36.8	1.4
VEGETABLES				
Asparagus	4 spears	13	3.5	2.9
Beets	1 cup	75	16.9	3.4
Broccoli	1 cup	55	5.8	2.3
Brussels sprouts	1 cup	56	11	4.1
Cabbage	1 cup	17	3.9	1.6
Carrots	1 carrot	30	10.5	3.1
Cauliflower	1 cup	25	5.3	2.5
Celery	1 cup	17	3.6	1.9

Item	Amount	Calories	Carb grams	Fiber grams
Collard greens	1 cup	92	9	5.3
Corn	1 cup	133	31.7	3.9
Cucumbers	1 cup	16	3.8	0.8
Eggplant	1 cup	28	7	2.5
Endive	1 cup	9	2	1.6
Kale	1 cup	39	7	2.6
Leeks	1 cup	32	8	1
Lettuce, iceberg	1 cup	8	1.6	0.7
Lima beans	1 cup	170	32	9.9
Mushrooms	1 cup	15	2.3	0.8
Mustard greens	1 cup	21	3	2.8
Okra	1 cup	52	11	5.2
Onions	1 cup	67	16.2	2.2
Parsnips	1 cup	111	26.5	5.6
Potato w/ skin	1	118	27.4	2.4
Peas	1 cup	125	22.8	8.8
Peppers, green	1 cup	30	6.9	2.5
Radishes	1 radish	1	0.2	0.1
Red hot chili pepper	1	18	4	0.7
Romaine lettuce	1 cup	10	1.8	1.2
Soybeans	1 cup	254	20	7.6
Scallions	1 cup	32	7.3	2.6
Spinach	1 cup	7	1.1	0.7
Squash, summer	1 cup	18	3.8	2.5
Squash, winter	1 cup	76	18.1	2.5
Sweet potato	1	131	30.2	4.8
Tomatoes	1 cup	32	7.1	2.2
Turnips	1 cup	34	7.9	3.1
Water chestnuts	1 cup	70	17.2	3.5

Glycemic Loads of Common Foods

The glycemic load (GL) is a scale used to indicate how much one serving of a particular food raises a person's blood sugar. A GL of 10 or less is considered low. Check your blood sugar two hours after eating a food to find out how it affects your blood sugar, since your reaction might be different. The GL is closely tied to portion size; if you eat twice as much as the portion size indicated, the food will have double the effect on your blood sugar. (Keep in mind that these portion sizes aren't necessarily the same as those used in the diabetic exchange system.) Work with your registered dietitian to figure out how to fit more low-GL foods into your eating plan.

LOW (GL = 10 OR LESS)

Breads, Tortillas, Grains	Serving size	GL
Coarse barley bread (75% intact kernels)	2 slices	10
Soy and flaxseed bread	2 slices	10
Whole-grain pumpernickel bread	2 slices	10
Pearled barley	1 cup	8
Popcorn	2 cups	8
Wheat tortillas	2 6-inch	6

Breakfast Cereals	Serving size	GL
Alpen Muesli	⅓ cup (1 oz.)	10
Oatmeal, instant 1 cup prepared	(1 oz.)	10
All-Bran	½ cup (1 oz.)	9
Bran Buds	⅓ cup (1 oz.)	7
Oatmeal from rolled oats	1 cup prepared (1 oz.)	7

Beans and Peas	Serving size	GL
Lima beans	1 cup	10
Pinto beans	1 cup	10
Chickpeas	1 cup	8
Baked beans	1 cup	7
Kidney beans	1 cup	7
Navy beans	1 cup	7
Butter beans	1 cup	6
Green peas	1 cup	6
Split peas, yellow	1 cup	6
Lentils, green or red	1 cup	5

Dairy and Soy Drinks	Serving size	GL
Low-fat yogurt with fruit and sugar	7 oz.	9
Soy milk	1 cup (8 oz.)	7
Low-fat chocolate milk, sweetened with aspartame	1 cup (8 oz.)	3
Low-fat yogurt with fruit, sweetened with aspartame	7 oz.	2

Fruits and Vegetables	Serving size	GL
Prunes, pitted, chopped	⅓ cup (2 oz.)	10
Apricots, dried, chopped	⅓ cup (2 oz.)	9
Peaches, canned in light syrup	½ cup (4 oz.)	9
Grapes, medium bunch	about 50 (4 oz.)	8
Mango, sliced	⅔ cup (4 oz.)	8
Pineapple, diced	⅔ cup (4 oz.)	7
Apple	1 small	6
Kiwifruit, sliced	⅔ cup (4 oz.)	6
Beets, sliced	½ cup	5
Orange	1 small	5
Peach	1 small	5
Plums	2 small	5
Pear	1 small	4
Strawberries	about 6 medium	4
Watermelon, chopped	⅔ cup (4 oz.)	4
Carrots, raw	1 large	3
Cherries	about 16 (4 oz.)	3
Grapefruit	½	3

Beverages	Serving size	GL
Orange juice, unsweetened	¾ cup (6 oz.)	10
Grapefruit juice, unsweetened	¾ cup (6 oz.)	7
Tomato juice	¾ cup (6 oz.)	4

Sweets	Serving size	GL
M&Ms with peanuts	25 (1 oz.)	6
Nutella (chocolate hazelnut spread)	4 Tbsp.	4

Nuts	Serving size	GL
Mixed nuts, roasted	⅓ cup (1.5 oz.)	4
Cashew nuts	about 13 (1.5 oz.)	3
Peanuts	⅓ cup (1.5 oz.)	1

MEDIUM (GL = 11–19)

Bread, Tortillas, Crackers, Chips	Serving size	GL
Coarse barley bread (50% intact kernels)	2 slices	18
High-fiber white bread	2 slices	18
Corn chips	2 oz.	17
100% whole-grain bread	2 slices	14
Sourdough rye bread	2 slices	12
Stone-ground wheat thins	4	12
Corn tortillas	2 6-inch	11

Grains	Serving size	GL
Converted long-grain white rice	²/₃ cup cooked	16
Brown rice	²/₃ cup cooked	18
Quinoa	²/₃ cup cooked	16
Wild rice	²/₃ cup cooked	18
Bulgur	²/₃ cup cooked	12

Pasta	Serving size	GL
Spaghetti (cooked 15 minutes)	1 cup	17
Whole-wheat spaghetti	1 cup	13
High-protein spaghetti	1 cup	12

Beverages	Serving size	GL
Low-fat chocolate milk	8 oz.	12
Pineapple juice, unsweetened	6 oz.	12
Apple juice	8 oz.	8

Fruits, Vegetables, Beans	Serving size	GL
Sweet corn	1 cup	18
Sweet potato	1 medium (5 oz.)	17
Figs, dried, chopped	¹/₃ cup (2 oz.)	16
Banana	1 small (4 oz.)	11
Black-eyed peas	1 cup	11

Breakfast Cereals	Serving size	GL
Nabisco Cream of Wheat, regular	1 cup prepared (1 oz.)	17
Post Grape-Nuts	½ cup (1 oz.)	16
Cheerios	1 cup (1 oz.)	15
Life	¾ cup (1 oz.)	15
Special K	1 cup (1 oz.)	14

HIGH (GL = 20 OR HIGHER)

Potatoes	Serving size	GL
Baked russet Burbank potato	1 medium	26
French fries	5 oz.	22

Grains	Serving size	GL
Sticky white rice	²/₃ cup cooked	31
Couscous	²/₃ cup cooked	23
Long-grain white rice	²/₃ cup cooked	23

Pasta	Serving size	GL
Udon Japanese noodles	1 cup cooked	25
Spaghetti (cooked 20 minutes)	1 cup	22

Breads	Serving size	GL
French baguette	2 slices	30
Middle Eastern flatbread	1 large	30
Italian white bread	2 slices	22
Hamburger roll	1	21
Mini-bagel (Lender's)	1	20
Wonder Bread	2 slices	20

Breakfast Cereals	Serving size	GL
Kellogg's Cornflakes	1 cup (1 oz.)	24
Rice Chex	1¼ cups (1 oz.)	23
Nabisco Cream of Wheat, instant	1 cup prepared (1 oz.)	22
Rice Krispies	¾ cup (1 oz.)	22
Corn Chex	1 cup (1 oz.)	21

Dried Fruit	Serving size	GL
Raisins	¹/₃ cup	28
Dates, dried, chopped	¹/₃ cup	25

Beverages	Serving size	GL
Ocean Spray Cranberry Juice Cocktail	12 oz.	36
Coca-Cola	12 oz.	24

Sweets	Serving size	GL
Mars Bar	2 oz.	26
Jelly beans	20	22

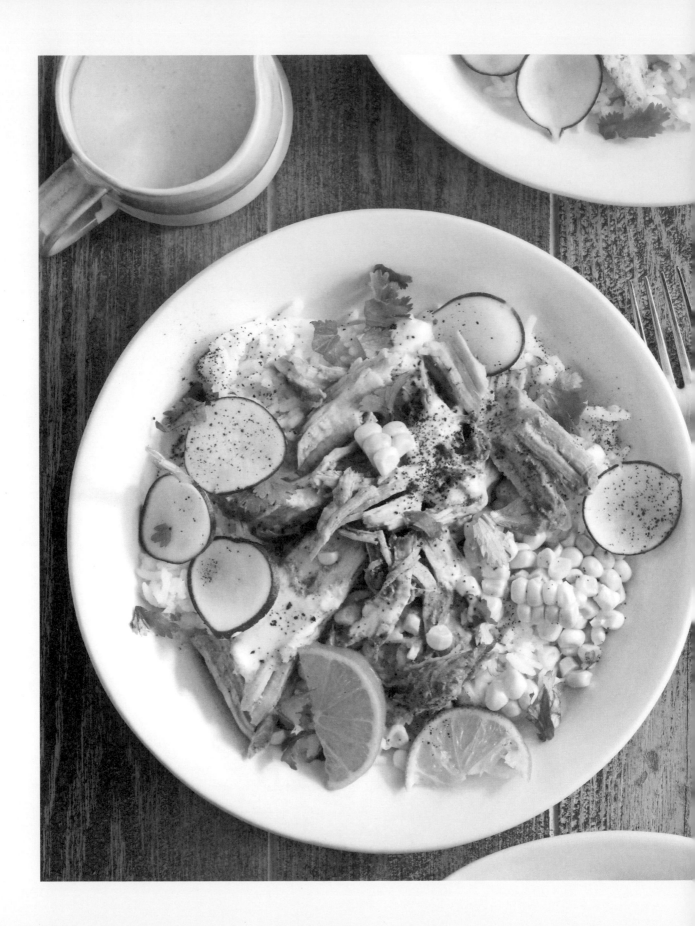

6

Reverse Diabetes
RECIPES

- Easy-to-Make Meals
- Diabetes-Friendly Dishes
- Full-of-Flavor Nutrition

Get Ready to Eat Well

WHAT YOU EAT IS, of course, a key component of your Reverse Diabetes plan. To help you meet your Eat goals, we've included more than 60 diabetes-friendly recipes here for you that are chock-full of fruits and vegetables, include lean protein and heart-healthy fats, replace refined carbohydrates with fiber-rich whole grains and legumes, and are relatively low in added sugars and salt. Best of all, they're delicious and easy to make.

That being said, there's always room for improvement. Here are some ideas on how you can make these nourishing recipes even more healthy.

Make them meatless. Where you can, swap out the meat in these recipes for plant-based proteins such as mushrooms, soy foods and beans. For instance, try extra-firm tofu cubes instead of chicken in the **Hearty Chicken Gyros** on page 209. Or TVP (textured vegetable protein) crumbles made of soy in place of the sausage and ground beef in the **Italian Mushroom Meatloaf** on page 223.

Reduce sodium. While people with diabetes tend to pay more attention to sugar than salt content, you should also keep sodium in check. Look for reduced-sodium or no-salt-added versions any time you use canned or jarred beans, vegetables, or sauce (such as in the **Beef & Bulgur-Stuffed Zucchini Boats** on page 216). Rinse them in water several times before adding them into the recipe. Replace deli meats such as those in the **Deli Turkey Lettuce Wraps** on page 206 with grilled chicken breast without added salt.

At the end of this chapter, you'll find six sample meal plans to give you an idea of what balanced nutrition throughout the day might look. Three of them incorporate recipes we've provided, in some cases pairing them with a simple side dish or beverage. We understand that you won't necessarily want to cook this much in a given day, which is totally fine. The plans are not necessarily intended to be followed exactly as written—feel free to mix and match meals to suit your needs and taste buds.

Plant-Based "Meats"

As plant-forward eating has become more popular, the food industry has responded with a plethora of plant-based "meats." Nutritionally speaking, however, not all meat alternatives are created equal. Look for options with a limited number of ingredients that also provide at least 10 to 15g of protein per serving and are comparatively low in sodium, fats, and filler carbs such as tapioca starch and powdered rice.

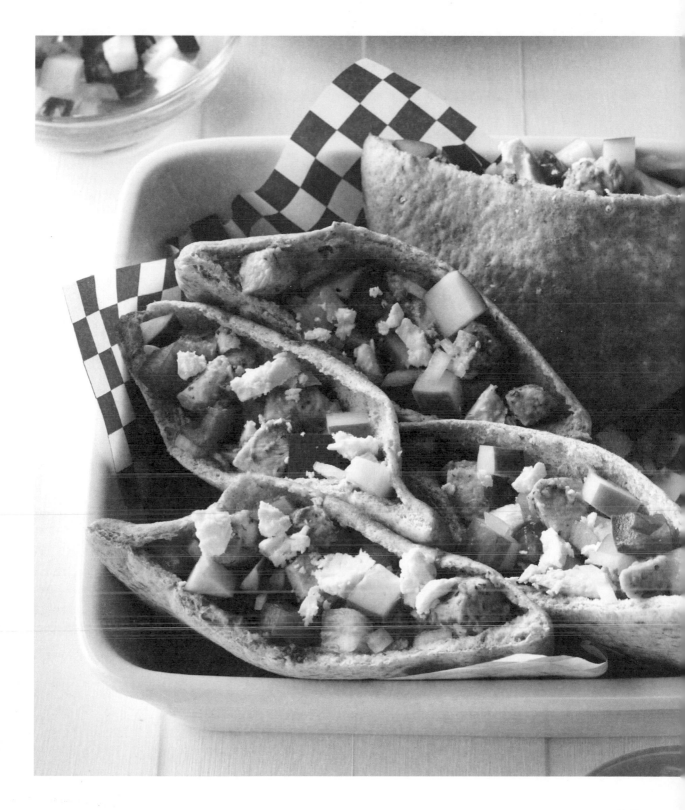

Breakfasts

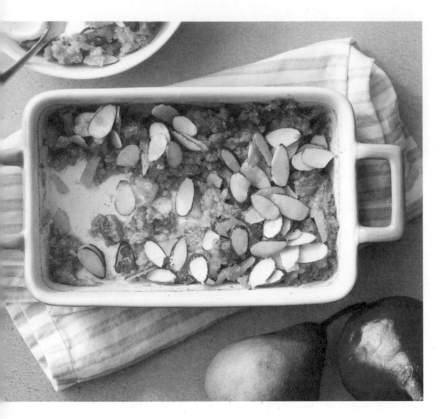

Turkey Sausage Patties

Serves 6

2 to 3 tsp. rubbed sage
1 tsp. brown sugar
¼ tsp. crushed red pepper flakes
¼ tsp. ground nutmeg
¼ tsp. pepper
Pinch allspice
1 lb. lean ground turkey

- **ONE** In a bowl, combine the first 6 ingredients. Add turkey; mix lightly but thoroughly. Shape into 6 patties.

- **TWO** Lightly coat a skillet with cooking spray. Cook patties over medium heat until browned on both sides and the meat is no longer pink, 15-20 minutes.

1 patty: 117 cal., 6g fat (2g sat. fat), 60mg chol., 71mg sod., 1g carb. (1g sugars, 0 fiber), 13g pro. *Diabetic exchanges:* 2 lean meat.

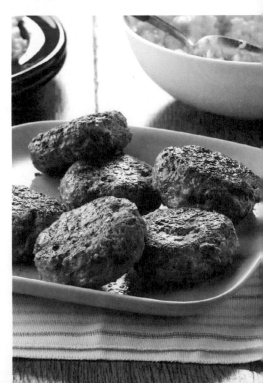

Pear Quinoa Breakfast Bake

Serves 2

1 cup water
¼ cup quinoa, rinsed
¼ cup mashed peeled ripe pear
1 Tbsp. honey
¼ tsp. ground cinnamon
¼ tsp. vanilla extract
Dash ground ginger
Dash ground nutmeg

Topping

¼ cup sliced almonds
1 Tbsp. brown sugar
1 Tbsp. butter, softened
Plain Greek yogurt, optional

- **ONE** Preheat the oven to 350°. In a small bowl, combine first 8 ingredients; transfer to a greased 3-cup baking dish. Cover and bake for 50 minutes. In another bowl, combine the almonds, brown sugar and butter; sprinkle over quinoa mixture.

- **TWO** Bake, uncovered, until lightly browned, 5-10 minutes longer. Let stand 10 minutes before serving. If desired, serve with yogurt.

1 serving: 267 cal., 13g fat (4g sat. fat), 15mg chol., 49mg sod., 35g carb. (18g sugars, 4g fiber), 6g pro. *Diabetic exchanges:* 2½ fat, 2 starch.

Muffin-Tin Scrambled Eggs

Makes 2 dozen

24	large eggs
1	tsp. salt
½	tsp. pepper
¼	tsp. garlic powder
1	jar (4 oz.) sliced mushrooms, finely chopped
1	can (4 oz.) chopped green chiles
3	oz. sliced deli ham, finely chopped
½	medium onion, finely chopped
½	cup shredded cheddar cheese
	Pico de gallo, optional

● **ONE** Preheat oven to 350°. In a large bowl, whisk eggs, salt, pepper and garlic powder until blended. Stir in mushrooms, chiles, ham, onion and cheese. Spoon about ¼ cup mixture into each of 24 greased muffin cups.

● **TWO** Bake 18-20 minutes or until eggs are set, rotating pans halfway through baking. Let stand 10 minutes before removing from pans. If desired, serve with pico de gallo.

1 egg cup: 88 cal., 6g fat (2g sat. fat), 190mg chol., 257mg sod., 1g carb. (0 sugars, 0 fiber), 8g pro. *Diabetic exchanges:* 1 medium-fat meat.

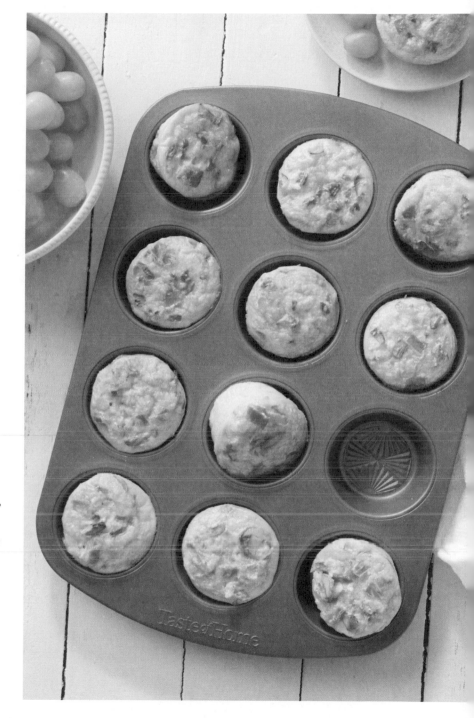

Breakfasts

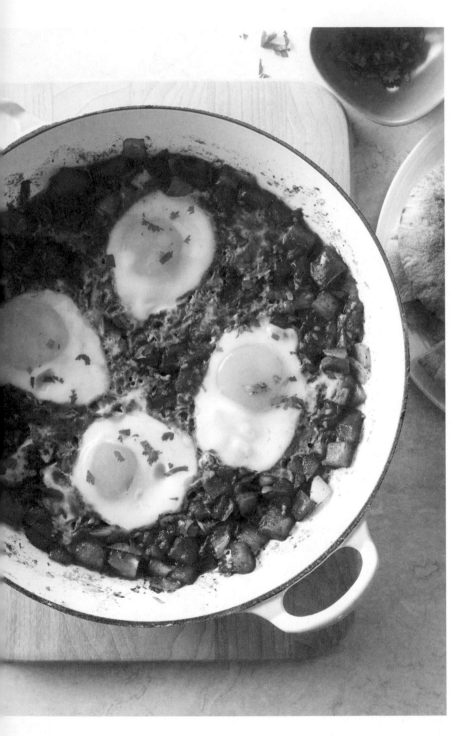

Shakshuka
Serves 4

- 2 Tbsp. olive oil
- 1 medium onion, chopped
- 1 garlic clove, minced
- 1 tsp. ground cumin
- 1 tsp. pepper
- ½ to 1 tsp. chili powder
- ½ tsp. salt
- 1 tsp. Sriracha chili sauce or hot pepper sauce, optional
- 2 medium tomatoes, chopped
- 4 large eggs
  Chopped fresh cilantro
  Whole pita breads, toasted

- **ONE** In a large cast-iron or other heavy skillet, heat oil over medium heat. Add onion; cook and stir until tender, 4-6 minutes. Add garlic, seasonings and, if desired, chili sauce; cook 30 seconds longer. Add tomatoes; cook until mixture is thickened, stirring occasionally, 3-5 minutes.

- **TWO** With back of spoon, make 4 wells in vegetable mixture; break an egg into each well. Cook, covered, until egg whites are completely set and yolks begin to thicken but are not hard, 4-6 minutes. Sprinkle with cilantro; serve with pita bread.

1 serving: 159 cal., 12g fat (3g sat. fat), 186mg chol., 381mg sod., 6g carb. (3g sugars, 2g fiber), 7g pro. **Diabetic exchanges:** 1½ fat, 1 vegetable, 1 medium-fat meat.

Whole Wheat Pancakes

Makes 20 pancakes

- 2 cups whole wheat flour
- ½ cup toasted wheat germ
- 1 tsp. baking soda
- ½ tsp. salt
- 2 large eggs, room temperature
- 3 cups buttermilk
- 1 Tbsp. canola oil

- **ONE** In a large bowl, combine the flour, wheat germ, baking soda and salt. In another bowl, whisk the eggs, buttermilk and oil. Stir into dry ingredients just until blended.

- **TWO** Pour batter by ¼ cupfuls onto a hot griddle coated with cooking spray; turn when bubbles form on top. Cook until the pancake's second side is golden brown.

2 pancakes: 157 cal., 4g fat (1g sat. fat), 45mg chol., 335mg sod., 24g carb. (4g sugars, 4g fiber), 9g pro. *Diabetic exchanges:* 1½ starch, 1 fat.

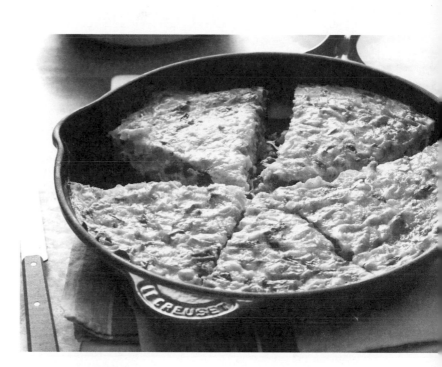

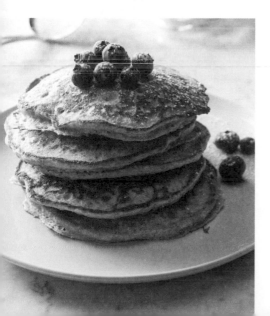

Colorful Pepper Frittata

Serves 6

- 4 large eggs
- 8 large egg whites
- 1 tsp. salt
- ½ tsp. pepper
- 1 cup shredded part-skim mozzarella cheese
- ¼ cup minced fresh basil
- 2 tsp. canola oil
- 1 large onion, chopped
- 2 cups chopped sweet red peppers
- 1 cup chopped sweet yellow pepper
- 1 cup chopped sweet orange pepper
- 3 garlic cloves, minced
- 2 Tbsp. shredded Parmesan cheese

- **ONE** Preheat the oven to 350°. Whisk together first 4 ingredients. Stir in the mozzarella cheese and basil.

- **TWO** In a 10-in. cast-iron or other ovenproof skillet, heat oil over medium heat. Add onion; cook and stir 2 minutes. Add peppers; cook and stir until tender, 3-4 minutes. Stir in garlic; cook 1 minute.

- **THREE** Pour in egg mixture; remove from heat. Sprinkle with Parmesan cheese. Bake, uncovered, until eggs are completely set, 20-25 minutes. Let stand 5 minutes. Cut into wedges.

1 wedge: 188 cal., 9g fat (4g sat. fat), 137mg chol., 672mg sod., 11g carb. (6g sugars, 2g fiber), 16g pro. *Diabetic exchanges:* 2 medium-fat meat, 1 vegetable.

201

Breakfasts

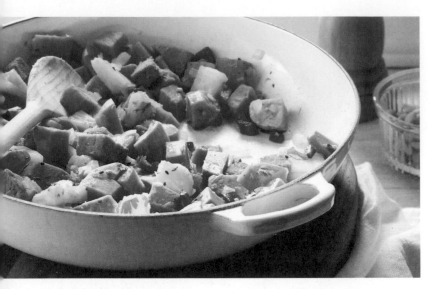

Hawaiian Hash
Serves 6

- 2 tsp. canola oil
- 1 tsp. sesame oil
- 4 cups cubed peeled sweet potatoes (about 1 lb.)
- 1 cup chopped onion
- ½ cup chopped sweet red pepper
- 1 tsp. minced fresh gingerroot
- ¼ cup water
- 1 cup cubed fully cooked ham
- 1 cup cubed fresh pineapple or unsweetened pineapple tidbits, drained
- ¼ cup salsa verde
- 1 tsp. soy sauce
- ½ tsp. black sesame seeds
  Chopped fresh cilantro
  Chopped macadamia nuts, optional

● **ONE** In a large cast-iron or other heavy skillet, heat oils over medium-high heat. Add sweet potatoes, onion, pepper and gingerroot; cook and stir 5 minutes. Add water. Reduce heat to low; cook, covered, until potatoes are tender, 8-10 minutes, stirring occasionally.

● **TWO** Stir in next 5 ingredients; cook and stir over medium-high heat until heated through, about 2 minutes. Top servings with cilantro and, if desired, chopped macadamia nuts.

¾ cup: 158 cal., 4g fat (1g sat. fat), 14mg chol., 440mg sod., 26g carb. (8g sugars, 4g fiber), 7g pro. *Diabetic exchanges:* 1½ starch, 1 lean meat, ½ fat.

French Omelet
Serves 2

- 2 large eggs, room temperature
- 4 large egg whites, room temperature
- ¼ cup fat-free milk
- ⅛ tsp. salt
- ⅛ tsp. pepper
- ¼ cup cubed fully cooked ham
- 1 Tbsp. chopped onion
- 1 Tbsp. chopped green pepper
- ¼ cup shredded reduced-fat cheddar cheese

● **ONE** Whisk together first 5 ingredients.

● **TWO** Place a 10-in. skillet coated with cooking spray over medium he at. Pour in egg mixture. Mixture should set immediately at edges. As eggs set, push cooked portions toward the center, letting uncooked eggs flow underneath. When eggs are thickened and no liquid egg remains, top 1 half with remaining ingredients. Fold omelet in half. Cut in half to serve.

½ omelet: 186 cal., 9g fat (4g sat. fat), 207mg chol., 648mg sod., 4g carb. (3g sugars, 0 fiber), 22g pro. *Diabetic exchanges:* 3 lean meat, 1 fat.

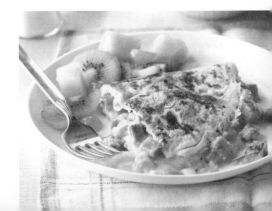

Portobello Mushrooms Florentine

Serves 2

- 2 large portobello mushrooms, stems removed
  Cooking spray
- ⅛ tsp. garlic salt
- ⅛ tsp. pepper
- ½ tsp. olive oil
- 1 small onion, chopped
- 1 cup fresh baby spinach
- 2 large eggs
- ⅛ tsp. salt
- ¼ cup crumbled goat cheese or feta cheese
  Minced fresh basil, optional

- **ONE** Preheat oven to 425°. Spritz mushrooms with cooking spray; place in a 15x10x1-in. pan, stem side up. Sprinkle with garlic salt and pepper. Bake, uncovered, until tender, about 10 minutes.

- **TWO** Meanwhile, in a nonstick skillet, heat oil over medium-high heat; saute onion until tender. Stir in spinach until wilted.

- **THREE** Whisk together eggs and salt; add to skillet. Cook and stir until eggs are thickened and no liquid egg remains; spoon onto mushrooms. Sprinkle with cheese and, if desired, basil.

1 stuffed mushroom: 126 cal., 5g fat (2g sat. fat), 18mg chol., 472mg sod., 10g carb. (4g sugars, 3g fiber), 11g pro. *Diabetic exchanges:* 2 vegetable, 1 lean meat, ½ fat.

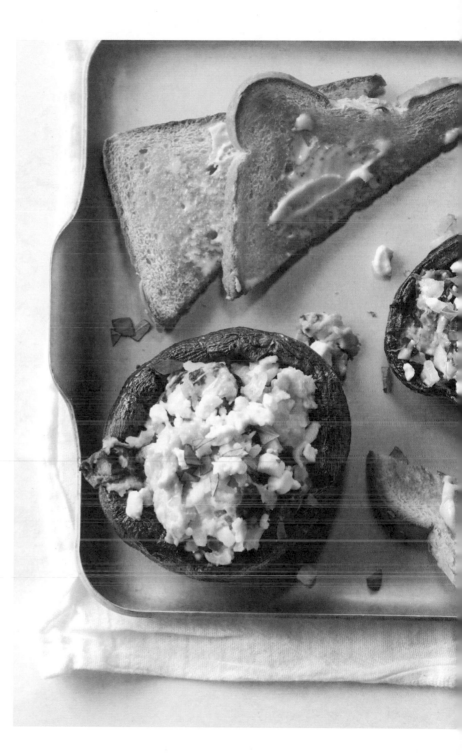

Breakfasts

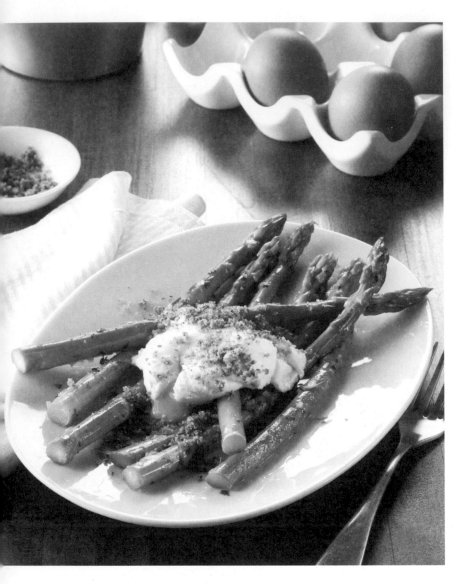

- **ONE** Place 3 in. of water in a large skillet with high sides; bring to a boil. Add asparagus; cook, uncovered, 2-4 minutes or until asparagus turns bright green. Remove asparagus and immediately drop into ice water. Drain and pat dry.

- **TWO** In a separate large skillet, heat oil over medium heat. Add garlic; cook and stir 1 minute. Add asparagus, tarragon, salt and pepper; cook asparagus 2-3 minutes or until crisp-tender, turning occasionally. Remove from pan; keep warm. In same skillet, melt butter over medium heat. Add bread crumbs; cook and stir 1-2 minutes or until toasted. Remove from heat.

- **THREE** Add 2-3 in. fresh water to skillet used to cook asparagus. Bring to a boil; adjust heat to maintain a gentle simmer. Break cold eggs, one at a time, into a small bowl; holding bowl close to surface of water, slip egg into water.

- **FOUR** Cook eggs, uncovered, 3-4 minutes or until whites are completely set and yolks begin to thicken but are not hard. Using a slotted spoon, lift eggs out of water; serve over asparagus. Sprinkle with toasted bread crumbs.

1 serving: 170 cal., 12g fat (4g sat. fat), 194mg chol., 513mg sod., 8g carb. (2g sugars, 1g fiber), 9g pro. ***Diabetic exchanges:*** 1½ fat, 1 vegetable, 1 medium-fat meat.

Poached Eggs with Tarragon Asparagus

Serves 4

- 1 lb. fresh asparagus, trimmed
- 1 Tbsp. olive oil
- 1 garlic clove, minced
- 1 Tbsp. minced fresh tarragon
- ½ tsp. salt
- ¼ tsp. pepper
- 1 Tbsp. butter
- ¼ cup seasoned bread crumbs
- 4 large eggs

Soups and Sandwiches

Tomato & Avocado Sandwiches

Serves 2

- ½ medium ripe avocado, peeled and mashed
- 4 slices whole wheat bread, toasted
- 1 medium tomato, sliced
- 2 Tbsp. finely chopped shallot
- ¼ cup hummus

● **SPREAD** avocado over 2 slices of toast. Top with tomato and shallot. Spread hummus over remaining toast slices; place on top of avocado toast, facedown on top of tomato layer.

1 sandwich: 278 cal., 11g fat (2g sat. fat), 0 chol., 379mg sod., 35g carb. (6g sugars, 9g fiber), 11g pro. ***Diabetic exchanges:*** 2 starch, 2 fat.

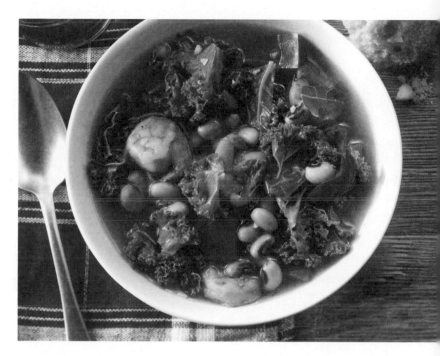

Carolina Shrimp Soup

Serves 6

- 4 tsp. olive oil, divided
- 1 lb. uncooked shrimp (31-40 per lb.), peeled and deveined
- 5 garlic cloves, minced
- 1 bunch kale, trimmed and coarsely chopped (about 16 cups)
- 1 medium sweet red pepper, cut into ¾-in. pieces
- 3 cups reduced-sodium chicken broth
- 1 can (15½ oz.) black-eyed peas, rinsed and drained
- ¼ tsp. salt
- ¼ tsp. pepper
  Minced fresh chives, optional

● **ONE** In a 6 qt. stockpot, heat 2 tsp. oil over medium-high heat. Add shrimp; cook and stir 2 minutes. Add garlic; cook just until shrimp turn pink, 1-2 minutes longer. Remove from pot.

● **TWO** In same pot, heat remaining 2 tsp. oil over medium-high heat. Stir in kale and red pepper; cook, covered, until kale is tender, stirring occasionally, 8-10 minutes. Add broth; bring to a boil. Stir in peas, salt, pepper and shrimp; heat through. If desired, sprinkle servings with chives.

1 cup: 188 cal., 5g fat (1g sat. fat), 92mg chol., 585mg sod., 18g carb. (2g sugars, 3g fiber), 19g pro. ***Diabetic exchanges:*** 2 lean meat, 2 vegetable, ½ starch, ½ fat.

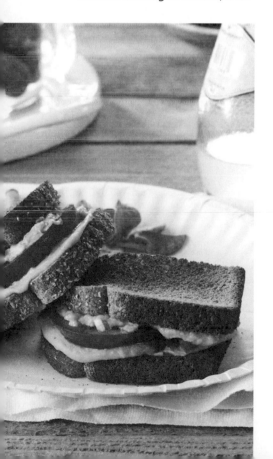

Soups and Sandwiches

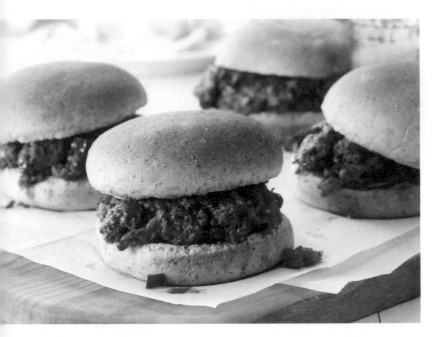

Beef & Veggie Sloppy Joes

Makes 10 sandwiches

- 4 medium carrots, shredded
- 1 medium yellow summer squash, shredded
- 1 medium zucchini, shredded
- 1 medium sweet red pepper, finely chopped
- 2 medium tomatoes, seeded and chopped
- 1 small red onion, finely chopped
- ½ cup ketchup
- 3 Tbsp. minced fresh basil or 3 tsp. dried basil
- 3 Tbsp. molasses
- 2 Tbsp. cider vinegar
- 2 garlic cloves, minced
- ½ tsp. salt
- ½ tsp. pepper
- 2 lbs. lean ground beef (90% lean)
- 10 whole wheat hamburger buns, split

- **ONE** In a 5- or 6-qt. slow cooker, combine the first 13 ingredients. In a large skillet, cook beef over medium heat until no longer pink, 8-10 minutes; crumble meat; drain. Transfer beef to slow cooker. Stir to combine.

- **TWO** Cook, covered, on low 5-6 hours or until heated through and vegetables are tender. Use a slotted spoon to serve beef mixture on buns.

1 sandwich: 316 cal., 10g fat (3g sat. fat), 57mg chol., 565mg sod., 36g carb. (15g sugars, 5g fiber), 22g pro. *Diabetic exchanges:* 2 starch, 2 lean meat, 1 vegetable.

Deli Turkey Lettuce Wraps

Makes 6 lettuce wraps

- 2 tsp. olive oil
- ½ medium red onion, thinly sliced
- 6 oz. sliced deli turkey, coarsely chopped
- 6 cherry tomatoes, halved
- 2 tsp. balsamic vinegar
- 6 Bibb or Boston lettuce leaves
- ½ medium ripe avocado, peeled and cubed
- ¼ cup shredded Swiss cheese
- ¼ cup alfalfa sprouts, optional

- **ONE** In a large skillet, heat oil over medium-high heat. Add onion; cook and stir until tender, 3-4 minutes. Add turkey; heat through. Stir in tomatoes and vinegar just until combined.

- **TWO** Serve in lettuce leaves. Top with avocado, cheese and, if desired, sprouts.

3 lettuce wraps: 270 cal., 16g fat (4g sat. fat), 43mg chol., 799mg sod., 11g carb. (4g sugars, 4g fiber), 22g pro. *Diabetic exchanges:* 3 lean meat, 1½ fat, 1 vegetable.

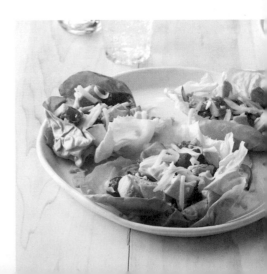

Yellow Squash Soup

Serves 8 (2 qt.)

- 2 large sweet onions, chopped
- 1 medium leek (white portion only), chopped
- 2 Tbsp. olive oil
- 6 garlic cloves, minced
- 6 medium yellow summer squash, seeded and cubed (about 6 cups)
- 4 cups reduced-sodium chicken broth
- 4 fresh thyme sprigs
- ¼ tsp. salt
- 2 Tbsp. lemon juice
- ⅛ tsp. hot pepper sauce
- 1 Tbsp. shredded Parmesan cheese
- 2 tsp. grated lemon zest

- **ONE** In a large saucepan, heat oil over medium heat. Add onions and leek; cook and stir until crisp-tender, 5 minutes. Add squash; cook and stir 5 minutes. Add garlic; cook and stir 1 minute longer. Stir in broth, thyme and salt. Bring to a boil. Reduce heat; cover and simmer until squash is tender, 15-20 minutes.

- **TWO** Discard thyme sprigs. Cool slightly. In a blender, process soup in batches until smooth. Return all to the pan. Stir in lemon juice and hot pepper sauce; heat through. Sprinkle each serving with cheese and lemon zest.

1 cup: 90 cal., 4g fat (1g sat. fat), 0 chol., 377mg sod., 12g carb. (6g sugars, 3g fiber), 4g pro. *Diabetic exchanges:* 1 starch, ½ fat.

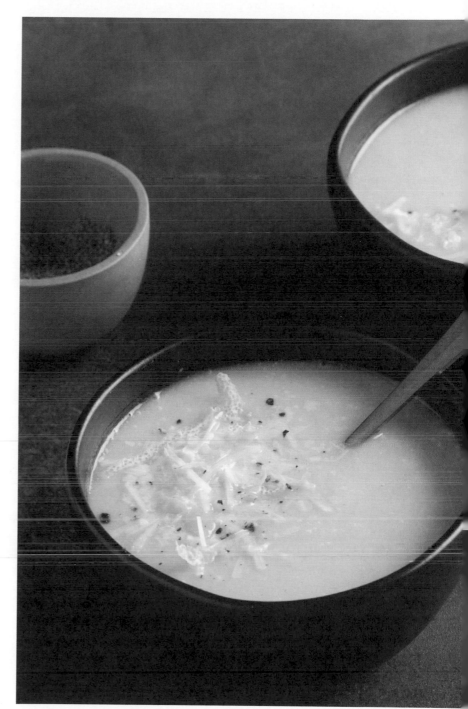

Soups and Sandwiches

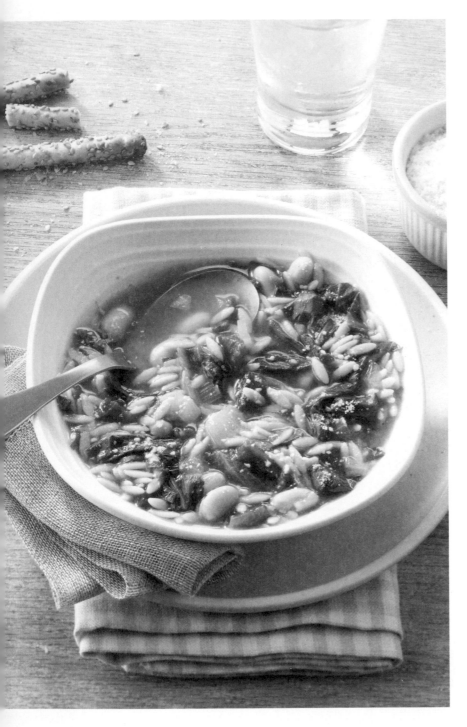

White Bean Soup with Escarole

Serves 8 (2 qt.)

- 1 Tbsp. olive oil
- 1 small onion, chopped
- 5 garlic cloves, minced
- 3 cans (14½ oz. each) reduced-sodium chicken broth
- 1 can (14½ oz.) diced tomatoes, undrained
- ½ tsp. Italian seasoning
- ¼ tsp. crushed red pepper flakes
- 1 cup uncooked whole wheat orzo pasta
- 1 bunch escarole or spinach, coarsely chopped (about 8 cups)
- 1 can (15 oz.) cannellini beans, rinsed and drained
- ¼ cup grated Parmesan cheese

- **ONE** In a Dutch oven, heat oil over medium heat. Add onion and garlic; cook and stir until tender. Add broth, tomatoes, Italian seasoning and pepper flakes; bring to a boil. Reduce heat; simmer, uncovered, 15 minutes.

- **TWO** Stir in orzo and escarole. Return to a boil; cook 12-14 minutes or until orzo is tender. Add beans; heat through, stirring occasionally. Sprinkle servings with cheese.

1 cup soup with 1½ tsp. cheese: 174 cal., 3g fat (1g sat. fat), 2mg chol., 572mg sod., 28g carb. (3g sugars, 8g fiber), 9g pro. **Diabetic exchanges:** 1 starch, 1 vegetable, 1 lean meat, ½ fat.

Butternut Squash & Barley Soup

Serves 12

- 1 small butternut squash (2½ to 3 lbs.), peeled and cut into 1-in. cubes (about 6 cups)
- 4 cups water
- 1 carton (32 oz.) reduced-sodium chicken broth
- ¾ cup medium pearl barley
- 2 medium carrots, chopped
- 2 celery ribs, chopped
- 1 small onion, chopped
- 2 Tbsp. minced fresh parsley or 2 tsp. dried parsley flakes
- 2 garlic cloves, minced
- 1 tsp. rubbed sage
- 1¼ tsp. salt
- ½ tsp. curry powder
- ¼ tsp. pepper
- 1 cup cubed cooked turkey

- **ONE** Place all ingredients except turkey in a 5- or 6-qt. slow cooker. Cook, covered, on low 5-7 hours or until squash and barley are tender.

- **TWO** Stir in turkey; cook, covered, about 15 minutes or until heated through.

1 cup: 120 cal., 1g fat (0 sat. fat), 12mg chol., 493mg sod., 23g carb. (4g sugars, 6g fiber), 7g pro. **Diabetic exchanges:** 1½ starch.

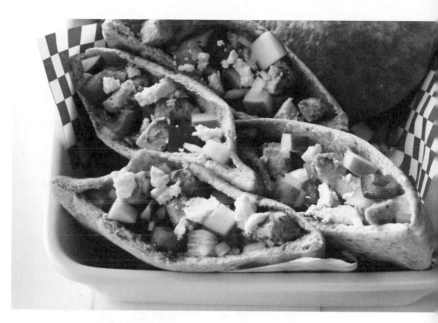

Hearty Chicken Gyros

Serves 6

- 1½ lbs. boneless skinless chicken breasts, cut into ½-in. cubes
- ½ cup salt-free lemon-pepper marinade
- 3 Tbsp. minced fresh mint

Sauce

- ½ cup fat-free plain Greek yogurt
- 2 Tbsp. lemon juice
- 1 tsp. dill weed
- ½ tsp. garlic powder

Assembly

- 1 medium cucumber, seeded and chopped
- 1 medium tomato, chopped
- ½ cup finely chopped onion
- 6 whole wheat pita pocket halves, warmed
- ⅓ cup crumbled feta cheese

- **ONE** Place chicken, marinade and mint in a shallow dish and turn to coat. Cover and refrigerate up to 6 hours.

- **TWO** Drain chicken, discarding marinade. Place a large nonstick skillet over medium-high heat. Add chicken; cook and stir until no longer pink, 4-6 minutes.

- **THREE** In a small bowl, mix sauce ingredients. In another bowl, combine cucumber, tomato and onion. Serve chicken in pita pockets with sauce, vegetable mixture and cheese.

1 gyro: 248 cal., 4g fat (2g sat. fat), 66mg chol., 251mg sod., 22g carb. (4g sugars, 3g fiber), 30g pro. **Diabetic exchanges:** 3 lean meat, 1½ starch, ½ fat.

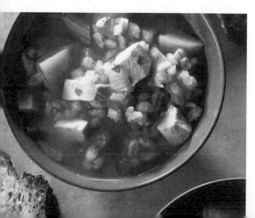

Soups and Sandwiches

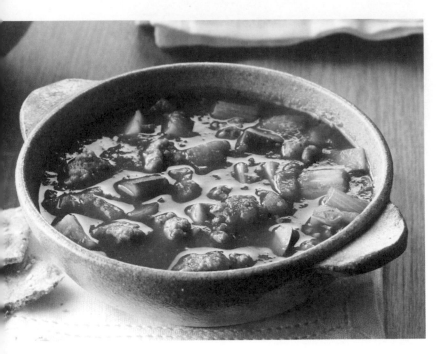

Italian Sausage Zucchini Soup

Serves 10 (3¼ qt.)

- 1 pkg. (19½ oz.) hot or sweet Italian turkey sausage links, casings removed
- 4 celery ribs, chopped
- 1 medium onion, chopped
- 2 tsp. Italian seasoning
- 1 tsp. dried oregano
- ½ tsp. salt
- ½ tsp. garlic powder
- ½ tsp. dried basil
- 2 medium zucchini, cut into ½-in. cubes
- 2 medium green peppers, chopped
- 4 cans (14½ oz. each) no-salt-added whole tomatoes, undrained, crushed
- 1 can (14½ oz.) reduced-sodium chicken broth
- 1 tsp. sugar

- **ONE** In a 6-qt. stockpot, cook and crumble sausage over medium-high heat until no longer pink, 5-7 minutes. Remove with a slotted spoon.

- **TWO** Add celery, onion and seasonings to same pot; cook and stir until onion is tender, 4-6 minutes. Stir in sausage and remaining ingredients; bring to a boil. Reduce heat; simmer, covered, until zucchini and peppers are tender, about 30 minutes.

1¼ cups: 104 cal., 4g fat (1g sat. fat), 20mg chol., 483mg sod., 10g carb. (6g sugars, 4g fiber), 9g pro. *Diabetic exchanges:* 1 lean meat, 1 vegetable.

Hearty Breaded Fish Sandwiches

Serves 4

- ½ cup dry bread crumbs
- ½ tsp. garlic powder
- ½ tsp. cayenne pepper
- ½ tsp. dried parsley flakes
- 4 cod fillets (6 oz. each)
- 4 whole wheat hamburger buns, split
- ¼ cup plain yogurt
- ¼ cup fat-free mayonnaise
- 2 tsp. lemon juice
- 2 tsp. sweet pickle relish
- ¼ tsp. dried minced onion
  Lettuce leaves, tomato slices and onion slices

- **ONE** In a shallow bowl, combine the bread crumbs, garlic powder, cayenne and parsley. Coat fillets.

- **TWO** On a lightly oiled grill rack, grill cod, covered, over medium heat for 4-5 minutes on each side or until fish flakes easily with a fork. Grill buns 30-60 seconds or until toasted.

- **THREE** In a small bowl, mix the yogurt, mayonnaise, lemon juice, relish and minced onion; spread over bun bottoms. Top with cod, lettuce, tomato and onion; replace bun tops.

1 sandwich: 292 cal., 4g fat (1g sat. fat), 68mg chol., 483mg sod., 32g carb. (7g sugars, 4g fiber), 32g pro. *Diabetic exchanges:* 5 lean meat, 2 starch.

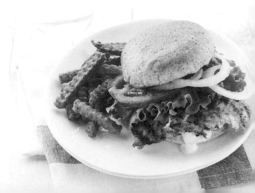

Main Meals

Strawberry-Blue Cheese Steak Salad

Serves 4

1	beef top sirloin steak (¾ in. thick and 1 lb.)
½	tsp. salt
¼	tsp. pepper
2	tsp. olive oil
2	Tbsp. lime juice

Salad

1	bunch romaine, torn (about 10 cups)
2	cups fresh strawberries, halved
¼	cup thinly sliced red onion
¼	cup crumbled blue cheese
¼	cup chopped walnuts, toasted
	Reduced-fat balsamic vinaigrette

● **ONE** Season steak with salt and pepper. In a large skillet, heat oil over medium heat. Add steak; cook 5-7 minutes on each side until meat reaches desired doneness (for medium-rare, a thermometer should read 135°; medium, 140°; medium-well, 145°). Remove from pan; let stand 5 minutes. Cut steak into bite-sized strips; toss with lime juice.

● **TWO** On a platter, combine romaine, strawberries and onion; top with steak. Sprinkle with cheese and walnuts. Serve with vinaigrette.

1 serving: 289 cal., 15g fat (4g sat. fat), 52mg chol., 452mg sod., 12g carb. (5g sugars, 4g fiber), 29g pro. *Diabetic exchanges:* 4 lean meat, 2 vegetable, 2 fat, ½ fruit.

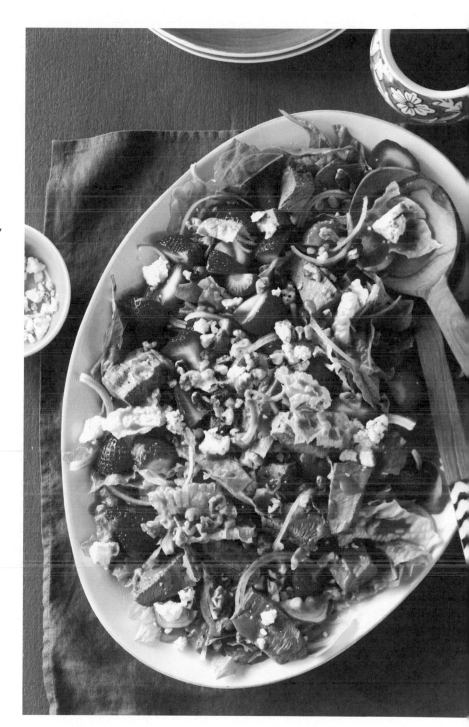

Main Meals

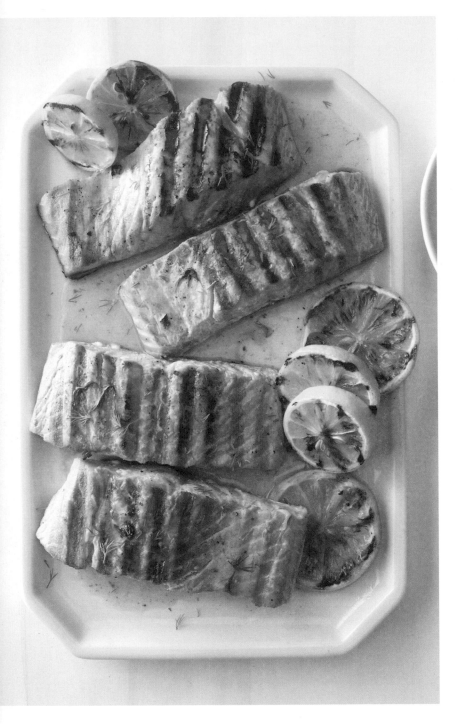

Lemony Grilled Salmon Fillets with Dill Sauce

Serves 4

- 2 medium lemons
- 4 salmon fillets (6 oz. each)

Lemon dill sauce

- 2½ tsp. cornstarch
- ½ cup water
- ⅓ cup lemon juice
- 4 tsp. butter
- 3 lemon slices, quartered
- 1 Tbsp. snipped fresh dill
- ¼ tsp. salt
- ⅛ tsp. dried chervil
  Dash cayenne pepper

● **ONE** Trim both ends from each lemon; cut lemons into thick slices. Grill salmon and lemon slices, covered, over high heat on an oiled grill rack or broil 3-4 in. from the heat for 3-5 minutes on each side or until the fish flakes easily with a fork and lemons are lightly browned.

● **TWO** For sauce, in a small saucepan, combine the cornstarch, water and lemon juice; add butter. Cook and stir over medium heat until thickened and bubbly. Remove from the heat; stir in quartered lemon slices and seasonings. Serve with salmon and grilled lemon slices.

1 fillet with 3 Tbsp. sauce: 320 cal., 20g fat (6g sat. fat), 97mg chol., 266mg sod., 6g carb. (1g sugars, 1g fiber), 29g pro. *Diabetic exchanges:* 3 lean meat, 1 fat.

Slow-Cooker Turkey Breast

Serves 14

- 1 bone-in turkey breast (6 to 7 lbs.), skin removed
- 1 Tbsp. olive oil
- 1 tsp. dried minced garlic
- 1 tsp. seasoned salt
- 1 tsp. paprika
- 1 tsp. Italian seasoning
- 1 tsp. pepper
- ½ cup water

- **BRUSH** turkey with oil. Combine the garlic, seasoned salt, paprika, Italian seasoning and pepper; rub over turkey. Transfer to a 6-qt. slow cooker; add water. Cover and cook on low for 5-6 hours or until tender.

4 oz. cooked turkey: 173 cal., 2g fat (0 sat. fat), 100mg chol., 171mg sod., 0 carb. (0 sugars, 0 fiber), 36g pro. **Diabetic exchanges:** 4 lean meat.

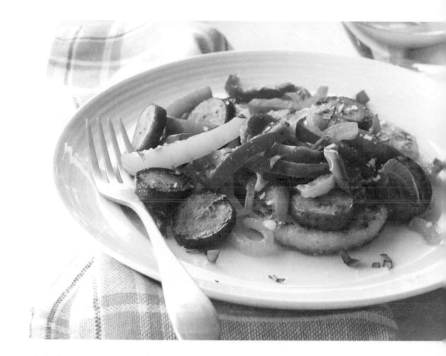

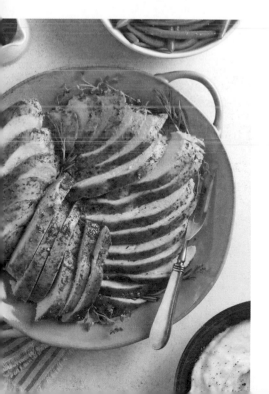

Chicken Sausages with Polenta

Serves 6

- 4 tsp. olive oil, divided
- 1 tube (1 lb.) polenta, cut into ½-in. slices
- 1 each medium green, sweet red and yellow peppers, thinly sliced
- 1 medium onion, thinly sliced
- 1 pkg. (12 oz.) fully cooked Italian chicken sausage links, thinly sliced
- ¼ cup grated Parmesan cheese
- 1 Tbsp. minced fresh basil

- **ONE** In a large nonstick skillet, heat 2 tsp. oil over medium heat. Add polenta; cook 9-11 minutes on each side or until golden brown. Keep warm.

- **TWO** Meanwhile, in another large skillet, heat remaining oil over medium-high heat. Add peppers and onion; cook and stir until tender. Remove from pan.

- **THREE** Add sausages to same pan; cook and stir 4-5 minutes or until browned. Return pepper mixture to pan; heat through. Serve with polenta; sprinkle with cheese and basil.

⅔ cup sausage mixture with 2 slices polenta: 212 cal., 9g fat (2g sat. fat), 46mg chol., 628mg sod., 19g carb. (4g sugars, 2g fiber), 13g pro. **Diabetic exchanges:** 2 lean meat, 1 starch, 1 vegetable, ½ fat.

Main Meals

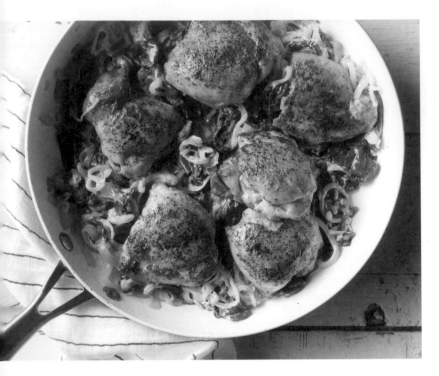

Chicken Thighs with Shallots & Spinach

Serves 6

- 6 boneless skinless chicken thighs (about 1½ lbs.)
- ½ tsp. seasoned salt
- ½ tsp. pepper
- 1½ tsp. olive oil
- 4 shallots, thinly sliced
- ⅓ cup white wine or reduced-sodium chicken broth
- 1 pkg. (10 oz.) fresh spinach, trimmed
- ¼ tsp. salt
- ¼ cup reduced-fat sour cream

- **ONE** Sprinkle chicken with seasoned salt and pepper. In a large nonstick skillet, heat oil over medium heat. Add chicken; cook until a thermometer reads 170°, about 6 minutes on each side. Remove from pan; keep warm.

- **TWO** In same pan, cook and stir shallots until tender. Add wine; bring to a boil. Cook until wine is reduced by half. Add spinach and salt; cook and stir just until spinach is wilted. Stir in sour cream; serve with chicken.

1 chicken thigh with ¼ cup spinach mixture: 223 cal., 10g fat (3g sat. fat), 77mg chol., 360mg sod., 7g carb. (2g sugars, 1g fiber), 23g pro. **Diabetic exchanges:** 3 lean meat, 1½ fat, 1 vegetable.

Greek Pork Chops

Serves 4

- 2 Tbsp. olive oil
- 4 tsp. lemon juice
- 1 Tbsp. Worcestershire sauce
- 2 tsp. dried oregano
- 1 tsp. salt
- 1 tsp. onion powder
- 1 tsp. garlic powder
- 1 tsp. pepper
- ½ tsp. ground mustard
- 4 boneless pork loin chops (¾ in. thick and 4 oz. each)

- **ONE** In a large bowl, mix first 9 ingredients. Add pork chops and turn to coat. Cover; refrigerate 8 hours or overnight.

- **TWO** Drain pork, discarding marinade. Grill chops, covered, over medium heat or broil 4 in. from heat until a thermometer reads 145°, 4-5 minutes per side. Let stand 5 minutes before serving.

1 pork chop: 193 cal., 10g fat (3g sat. fat), 55mg chol., 349mg sod., 2g carb. (0 sugars, 1g fiber), 22g pro. **Diabetic exchanges:** 3 lean meat, ½ fat.

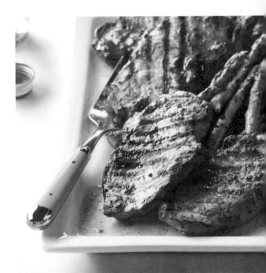

Chicken Florentine Meatballs

Serves 6

- 2 large eggs, lightly beaten
- 1 pkg. (10 oz.) frozen chopped spinach, thawed and squeezed dry
- ½ cup dry bread crumbs
- ¼ cup grated Parmesan cheese
- 1 Tbsp. dried minced onion
- 1 garlic clove, minced
- ¼ tsp. salt
- ⅛ tsp. pepper
- 1 lb. ground chicken
- 1 medium spaghetti squash

Sauce

- ½ lb. sliced fresh mushrooms
- 2 tsp. olive oil
- 1 can (14½ oz.) diced tomatoes, undrained
- 1 can (8 oz.) tomato sauce
- 2 Tbsp. minced fresh parsley
- 1 garlic clove, minced
- 1 tsp. dried oregano
- 1 tsp. dried basil

- **ONE** In a large bowl, combine the first eight ingredients. Crumble chicken over mixture and mix well. Shape into 1½-in. balls.

- **TWO** Place meatballs on a rack in a shallow baking pan. Bake, uncovered, at 400° for 20-25 minutes or until no longer pink. Meanwhile, cut squash in half lengthwise; discard seeds. Place squash cut side down on a microwave-safe plate. Microwave, uncovered, on high for 15-18 minutes or until tender.

- **THREE** For sauce, in a large nonstick skillet, saute mushrooms in oil until tender. Stir in the remaining ingredients. Bring to a boil. Reduce heat; simmer, uncovered, for 8-10 minutes or until slightly thickened. Add meatballs and heat through.

- **FOUR** When squash is cool enough to handle, use a fork to separate strands. Serve with meatballs and sauce.

1 serving: 303 cal., 12g fat (3g sat. fat), 123mg chol., 617mg sod., 31g carb. (4g sugars, 7g fiber), 22g pro. *Diabetic exchanges:* 3 lean meat, 2 starch, ½ fat.

Main Meals

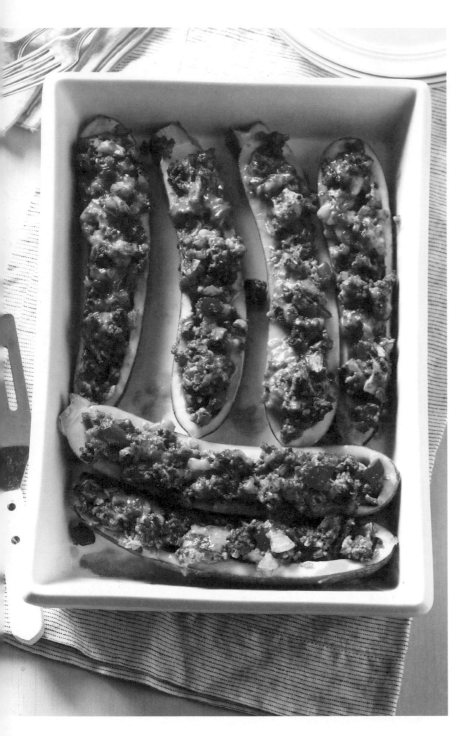

Beef & Bulgur-Stuffed Zucchini Boats

Serves 4

4	medium zucchini
1	lb. lean ground beef (90% lean)
1	large onion, finely chopped
1	small sweet red pepper, chopped
1½	cups tomato sauce
½	cup bulgur
¼	tsp. pepper
½	cup salsa
½	cup shredded reduced-fat cheddar cheese

- **ONE** Preheat oven to 350°. Cut each zucchini in half lengthwise. Scoop out flesh, leaving a ¼-in. shell; chop flesh.

- **TWO** In a large skillet, cook beef, onion and red pepper over medium heat 6-8 minutes or until meat is no longer pink, breaking it into crumbles; drain. Stir in tomato sauce, bulgur, pepper and zucchini flesh. Bring to a boil. Reduce heat; simmer, uncovered, 12-15 minutes or until bulgur is tender. Stir in salsa. Spoon into zucchini shells.

- **THREE** Place in a 13x9-in. baking dish coated with cooking spray. Bake, covered, 20 minutes. Sprinkle with cheese. Bake, uncovered, 10-15 minutes longer or until zucchini is tender and filling is heated through.

2 stuffed zucchini halves: 361 cal., 13g fat (6g sat. fat), 81mg chol., 714mg sod., 31g carb. (9g sugars, 7g fiber), 32g pro. *Diabetic exchanges:* 4 lean meat, 2 vegetable, 1 starch.

Red Pepper & Parmesan Tilapia

Serves 4

- 1 large egg, lightly beaten
- ½ cup grated Parmesan cheese
- 1 tsp. Italian seasoning
- ½ to 1 tsp. crushed red pepper flakes
- ½ tsp. pepper
- 4 tilapia fillets (6 oz. each)

● **ONE** Preheat oven to 425°. Place egg in a shallow bowl. In another shallow bowl, combine the cheese, Italian seasoning, pepper flakes and pepper. Dip fillets in egg and then in cheese mixture.

● **TWO** Place fillets in a 15x10x1-in. baking pan coated with cooking spray. Bake until fish just begins to flake easily with a fork, 10-15 minutes.

1 fillet: 179 cal., 4g fat (2g sat. fat), 89mg chol., 191mg sod., 1g carb. (0 sugars, 0 fiber), 35g pro. **Diabetic exchanges:** 5 very lean meat, ½ fat.

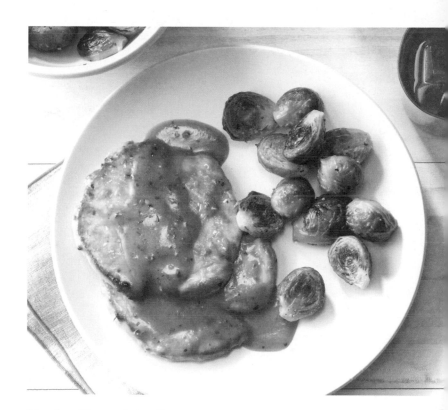

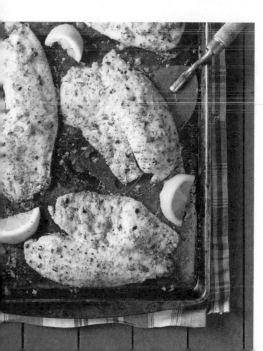

Herb-Glazed Turkey Slices

Serves 4

- 1 pkg. (17.6 oz.) turkey breast cutlets
- 1 Tbsp. canola oil
- ½ cup chicken broth
- ½ cup apple juice
- 1 Tbsp. honey
- 1 Tbsp. Dijon mustard
- ½ tsp. salt
- ¼ tsp. each dried basil, dried rosemary, crushed and garlic powder
- 1 Tbsp. cornstarch
- 1 Tbsp. water

● **ONE** In a large skillet, brown turkey slices on each side in oil. In a small bowl, combine the broth, apple juice, honey, mustard, salt, basil, rosemary and garlic powder; pour over turkey. Bring to a boil. Reduce heat; cover and simmer for 8 minutes or until the turkey is no longer pink.

● **TWO** Combine cornstarch and water until smooth; stir into skillet. Bring to a boil; cook and stir for 2 minutes or until thickened.

4 oz. cooked turkey: 213 cal., 4g fat (1g sat. fat), 78mg chol., 570mg sod., 11g carb. (8g sugars, 0 fiber), 31g pro. **Diabetic exchanges:** 4 lean meat, 1 fat, ½ starch.

Main Meals

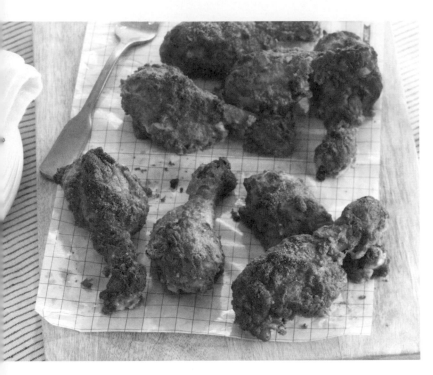

Oven-Fried Chicken Drumsticks

Serves 4

- 1 cup fat-free plain Greek yogurt
- 1 Tbsp. Dijon mustard
- 2 garlic cloves, minced
- 8 chicken drumsticks (4 oz. each), skin removed
- ½ cup whole wheat flour
- 1½ tsp. paprika
- 1 tsp. baking powder
- 1 tsp. salt
- 1 tsp. pepper
  Olive oil-flavored cooking spray

- **ONE** In a large bowl or dish, combine yogurt, mustard and garlic. Add chicken and turn to coat. Cover and refrigerate 8 hours or overnight.

- **TWO** Preheat oven to 425°. In another bowl, mix flour, paprika, baking powder, salt and pepper. Remove chicken from marinade and add, 1 piece at a time, to flour mixture; toss to coat. Place on a wire rack over a baking sheet; spritz with cooking spray. Bake 40-45 minutes or until a thermometer inserted into chicken reads 170°-175°.

2 chicken drumsticks: 227 cal., 7g fat (1g sat. fat), 81mg chol., 498mg sod., 9g carb. (2g sugars, 1g fiber), 31g pro. **Diabetic exchanges:** 4 lean meat, ½ starch.

Pork Chops with Dijon Sauce

Serves 4

- 4 boneless pork loin chops (6 oz. each)
- ¼ tsp. salt
- ¼ tsp. pepper
- 2 tsp. canola oil
- ⅓ cup reduced-sodium chicken broth
- 2 Tbsp. Dijon mustard
- ⅓ cup half-and-half cream

- **ONE** Sprinkle pork chops with salt and pepper. In a large skillet coated with cooking spray, brown chops in oil for 4-5 minutes on each side or until a thermometer reads 145°. Remove and keep warm.

- **TWO** Stir broth into skillet, scraping up any browned bits. Stir in mustard and half-and-half. Bring to a boil. Reduce heat; simmer, uncovered, until thickened, 5-6 minutes, stirring occasionally. Serve with pork chops.

1 pork chop: 283 cal., 14g fat (5g sat. fat), 92mg chol., 432mg sod., 1g carb. (1g sugars, 0 fiber), 34g pro. **Diabetic exchanges:** 5 lean meat, 2 fat.

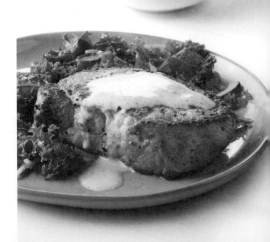

Fiery Stuffed Poblanos

Serves 8

- 8 poblano peppers
- 1 can (15 oz.) black beans, rinsed and drained
- 1 medium zucchini, chopped
- 1 small red onion, chopped
- 4 garlic cloves, minced
- 1 can (15¼ oz.) whole kernel corn, drained
- 1 can (14½ oz.) fire-roasted diced tomatoes, undrained
- 1 cup cooked brown rice
- 1 Tbsp. ground cumin
- 1 to 1½ tsp. ground ancho chile pepper
- ¼ tsp. salt
- ¼ tsp. pepper
- 1 cup shredded reduced-fat Mexican cheese blend, divided
- 3 green onions, chopped
- ½ cup reduced-fat sour cream

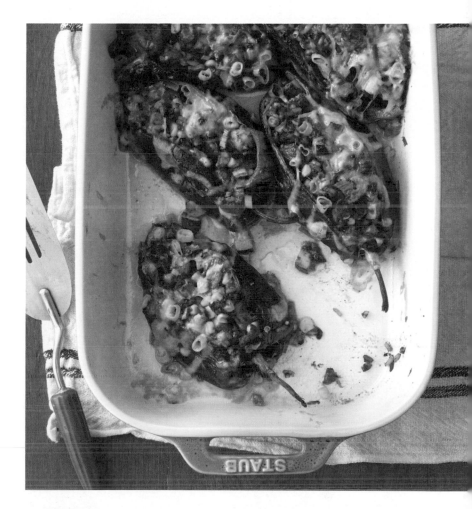

- **ONE** Broil peppers 3 in. from heat until skins blister, about 5 minutes. With tongs, rotate peppers a quarter turn. Broil and rotate until all sides are blistered and blackened. Immediately place peppers in a large bowl; cover and let stand for 20 minutes.

- **TWO** Meanwhile, in a small bowl, coarsely mash beans; set aside. In a large nonstick skillet, cook and stir zucchini and onion until tender. Add garlic; cook 1 minute longer. Add corn, tomatoes, rice, seasonings and beans. Remove from heat; stir in ½ cup cheese. Set aside.

- **THREE** Preheat oven to 375°. Peel charred skins from poblanos and discard. Cut a lengthwise slit through each pepper, leaving stem intact; discard membranes and seeds. Spoon ⅔ cup filling into each pepper.

- **FOUR** Place peppers in a 13x9-in. baking dish coated with cooking spray. Bake until heated through, 18-22 minutes, sprinkling with green onions and remaining cheese during last 5 minutes of baking. Serve with sour cream.

1 stuffed pepper: 223 cal., 5g fat (2g sat. fat), 15mg chol., 579mg sod., 32g carb. (9g sugars, 7g fiber), 11g pro. *Diabetic exchanges:* 2 vegetable, 1 starch, 1 lean meat, 1 fat.

Main Meals

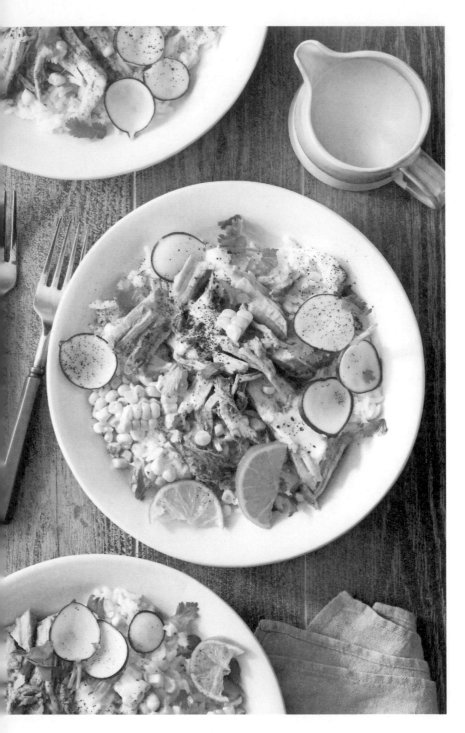

Slow-Cooker Al Pastor Bowls

Makes 8 cups

- 2 cans (7 oz. each) whole green chiles
- 1 can (20 oz.) pineapple chunks, drained
- 1 medium onion, chopped
- ½ cup orange juice
- ¼ cup white vinegar
- 3 garlic cloves, peeled
- 2 Tbsp. chili powder
- 2 tsp. salt
- 1½ tsp. smoked paprika
- 1 tsp. dried oregano
- 1 tsp. ground cumin
- ½ tsp. ground coriander
- 4 lbs. boneless pork loin roast
  Hot cooked rice
  Optional toppings: Black beans, chopped avocado, corn, sliced radishes, lime and Mexican crema

- **ONE** Puree first 12 ingredients in a blender. In a 5- or 6-qt. slow cooker, combine pork and pepper mixture. Cook, covered, on low until pork is very tender, 6-8 hours. Stir to break up pork.

- **TWO** Serve pork in bowls over rice. If desired, add toppings.

⅔ cup: 232 cal., 7g fat (3g sat. fat), 75mg chol., 512mg sod., 11g carb. (8g sugars, 1g fiber), 30g pro. *Diabetic exchanges:* 4 lean meat, ½ starch.

Cod & Asparagus Bake

Serves 4

- 4   cod fillets (4 oz. each)
- 1   lb. fresh thin asparagus, trimmed
- 1   pint cherry tomatoes, halved
- 2   Tbsp. lemon juice
- 1½ tsp. grated lemon zest
- ¼   cup grated Romano cheese

● **ONE** Preheat oven to 375°. Place cod and asparagus in a 15x10x1-in. baking pan brushed with oil. Add tomatoes, cut sides down. Brush fish with lemon juice; sprinkle with lemon zest. Sprinkle fish and vegetables with Romano cheese. Bake until fish just begins to flake easily with a fork, about 12 minutes.

● **TWO** Remove pan from oven; preheat broiler. Broil cod mixture 3-4 in. from heat until vegetables are lightly browned, 2-3 minutes.

1 serving: 141 cal., 3g fat (2g sat. fat), 45mg chol., 184mg sod., 6g carb. (3g sugars, 2g fiber), 23g pro. *Diabetic exchanges:* 3 lean meat, 1 vegetable.

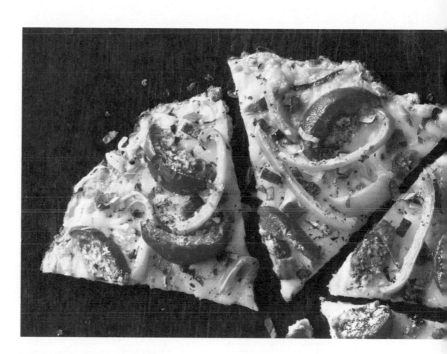

Zucchini Crust Pizza

Serves 6

- 2   cups shredded zucchini (1 to 1½ medium), squeezed dry
- ½   cup egg substitute or 2 large eggs, lightly beaten
- ¼   cup all-purpose flour
- ¼   tsp. salt
- 2   cups shredded part-skim mozzarella cheese, divided
- ⅓   cup grated Parmesan cheese, divided
- 2   small tomatoes, halved and sliced
- ½   cup chopped red onion
- ½   cup julienned bell pepper
- 1   tsp. dried oregano
- ½   tsp. dried basil Chopped fresh basil, optional

● **ONE** Preheat oven to 450°. In a large bowl, combine first 4 ingredients; stir in ½ cup mozzarella cheese and ¼ cup Parmesan cheese. Transfer to a 12-in. pizza pan coated generously with cooking spray; spread to an 11-in. circle.

● **TWO** Bake until golden brown, 13-16 minutes. Reduce oven setting to 400°. Sprinkle with remaining mozzarella cheese; top with tomatoes, onion, pepper, herbs and remaining Parmesan cheese. Bake until edge is golden brown and cheese is melted, 10-15 minutes. Sprinkle with chopped fresh basil, if desired.

1 piece: 188 cal., 10g fat (5g sat. fat), 30mg chol., 514mg sod., 12g carb. (4g sugars, 1g fiber), 14g pro. *Diabetic exchanges:* 2 lean meat, 2 vegetable, ½ fat.

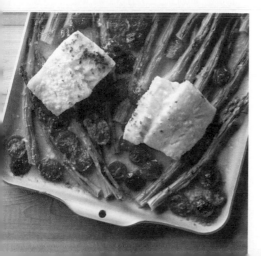

Main Meals

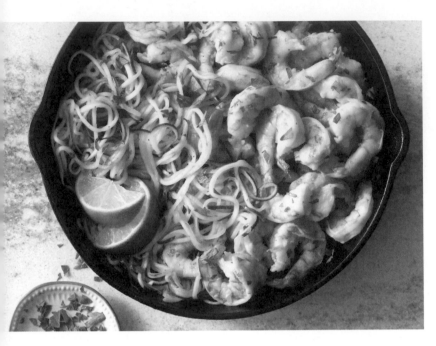

Tequila Lime Shrimp Zoodles

Serves 4

- 3 Tbsp. butter, divided
- 1 shallot, minced
- 2 garlic cloves, minced
- ¼ cup tequila
- 1½ tsp. grated lime zest
- 2 Tbsp. lime juice
- 1 Tbsp. olive oil
- 1 lb. uncooked shrimp (31-40 per lb.), peeled and deveined
- 2 medium zucchini, spiralized (about 6 cups)
- ½ tsp. salt
- ¼ tsp. pepper
- ¼ cup minced fresh parsley
  Additional grated lime zest

- **ONE** In a large cast-iron or other heavy skillet, heat 2 Tbsp. butter over medium heat. Add shallot and garlic; cook 1-2 minutes. Remove from heat; stir in tequila, lime zest and lime juice. Cook over medium heat until liquid is almost evaporated, 2-3 minutes.

- **TWO** Add olive oil and remaining butter; stir in shrimp and zucchini. Sprinkle with salt and pepper. Cook and stir until shrimp begin to turn pink and zucchini is crisp-tender, 4-5 minutes. Sprinkle with parsley and additional lime zest.

1¼ cups: 246 cal., 14g fat (6g sat. fat), 161mg chol., 510mg sod., 7g carb. (3g sugars, 1g fiber), 20g pro. ***Diabetic exchanges:*** 3 lean meat, 3 fat, 1 vegetable.

Balsamic Chicken with Roasted Tomatoes

Serves 4

- 2 Tbsp. honey
- 2 Tbsp. olive oil, divided
- 2 cups grape tomatoes
- 4 boneless skinless chicken breast halves (6 oz. each)
- ½ tsp. salt
- ½ tsp. pepper
- 2 Tbsp. balsamic glaze

- **ONE** Preheat oven to 400°. In a small bowl, mix honey and 1 Tbsp. oil. Add tomatoes and toss to coat. Transfer to a greased 15x10x1-in. baking pan. Bake 5-7 minutes or until softened.

- **TWO** Pound chicken breasts with a meat mallet to ½-in. thickness; sprinkle with salt and pepper. In a large skillet, heat remaining oil over medium heat. Add chicken; cook 5-6 minutes on each side or until no longer pink. Serve with roasted tomatoes; drizzle with glaze.

1 chicken breast half with ½ cup tomatoes and 1½ tsp. glaze: 306 cal., 11g fat (2g sat. fat), 94mg chol., 384mg sod., 16g carb. (14g sugars, 1g fiber), 35g pro. ***Diabetic exchanges:*** 5 lean meat, 1½ fat, 1 starch.

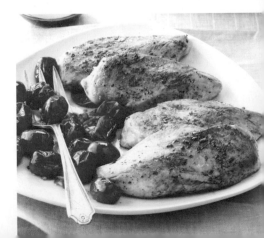

Italian Mushroom Meat Loaf

Serves 8

- 1 large egg, lightly beaten
- ¼ lb. fresh mushrooms, chopped
- ½ cup old-fashioned oats
- ½ cup chopped red onion
- ¼ cup ground flaxseed
- ½ tsp. pepper
- 1 pkg. (19½ oz.) Italian turkey sausage links, casings removed, crumbled
- 1 lb. lean ground beef (90% lean)
- 1 cup marinara or spaghetti sauce
  Shredded Parmesan cheese, optional

- **ONE** Preheat oven to 350°. In a large bowl, combine the egg, mushrooms, oats, onion, flax and pepper. Crumble turkey and beef over mixture; mix lightly but thoroughly.

- **TWO** Shape into a 10x4-in. loaf. Place in a 13x9-in. baking dish coated with cooking spray. Bake, uncovered, for 50 minutes; drain. Top with marinara sauce. Bake until no pink remains and a thermometer reads 160°, 10-15 minutes longer . If desired, top with Parmesan cheese.

1 slice: 261 cal., 14g fat (3g sat. fat), 103mg chol., 509mg sod., 10g carb. (3g sugars, 2g fiber), 25g pro. ***Diabetic exchanges:*** 3 lean meat, ½ starch.

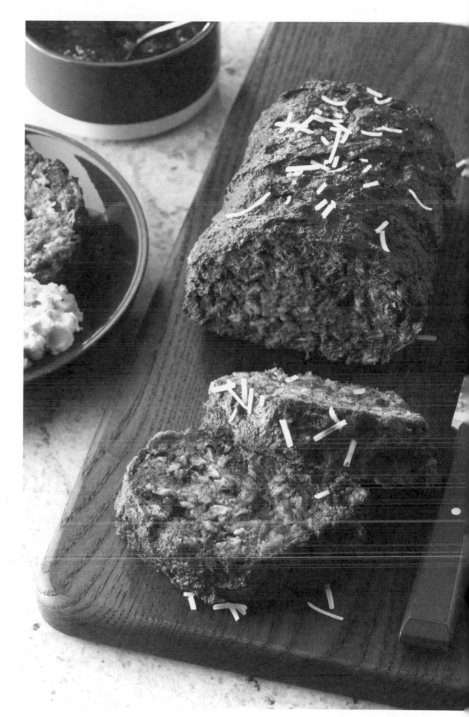

223

Main Meals

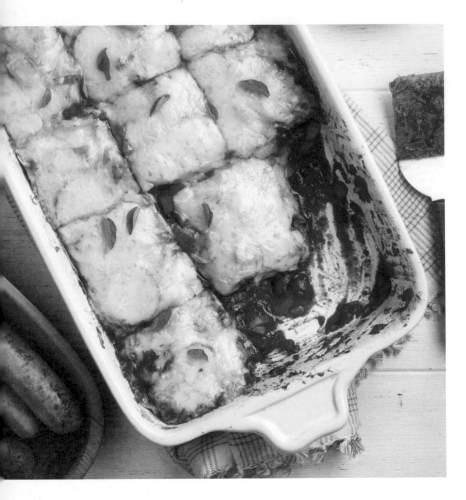

Easy Vegetable Lasagna

Serves 12

- 1 large onion, chopped
- 1 Tbsp. olive oil
- 6 garlic cloves, minced
- 1 can (28 oz.) tomato puree
- 1 can (8 oz.) tomato sauce
- 3 Tbsp. minced fresh basil
- 3 Tbsp. minced fresh oregano
- 1 tsp. sugar
- ½ tsp. crushed red pepper flakes

Roasted vegetables

- 4 cups sliced zucchini
- 3 cups sliced fresh mushrooms
- 2 medium green peppers, cut into 1-in. pieces
- 1 medium onion, cut into 1-in. pieces
- ½ tsp. salt
- ¼ tsp. pepper

- 6 lasagna noodles, cooked, rinsed and drained
- 4 cups shredded part-skim mozzarella cheese
- 1 cup shredded Parmesan cheese

● **ONE** Preheat oven to 450°. In a large saucepan, saute onion in oil until tender over medium heat; add garlic and cook 1 minute longer. Stir in the tomato puree, sauce and seasonings. Bring to a boil. Reduce heat; simmer, uncovered, until slightly thickened, 20-25 minutes.

● **TWO** Meanwhile, in a large bowl, combine the vegetables, salt and pepper. Transfer to two 15x10x1-in. baking pans coated with cooking spray. Bake until golden brown, 15-18 minutes. Reduce oven temperature to 400°.

● **THREE** Spread ½ cup of the sauce into a 13x9-in. baking dish coated with cooking spray. Layer with three noodles, 1¾ cups sauce, and half of the roasted vegetables and cheeses. Repeat layers.

● **FOUR** Cover and bake for 10 minutes. Uncover; bake until bubbly and golden brown, 10-15 minutes longer. Let stand for 10 minutes before serving. If desired, garnish with additional fresh oregano.

1 piece: 258 cal., 11g fat (6g sat. fat), 29mg chol., 571mg sod., 23g carb. (6g sugars, 3g fiber), 16g pro. *Diabetic exchanges:* 2 medium-fat meat, 2 vegetable, ½ starch.

Herbed Tuna & White Bean Salad

Serves 4

- 4 cups fresh arugula
- 1 can (15 oz.) no-salt-added cannellini beans, rinsed and drained
- 1 cup grape tomatoes, halved
- ½ small red onion, thinly sliced
- ⅓ cup chopped roasted sweet red peppers
- ⅓ cup pitted Nicoise or other olives
- ¼ cup chopped fresh basil
- 3 Tbsp. extra virgin olive oil
- ½ tsp. grated lemon zest
- 2 Tbsp. lemon juice
- 1 garlic clove, minced
- ⅛ tsp. salt
- 2 cans (5 oz. each) albacore white tuna in water, drained

- **PLACE** first 7 ingredients in a large bowl. Whisk together oil, lemon zest, lemon juice, garlic and salt; drizzle over salad. Add tuna and toss gently to combine.

2 cups: 319 cal., 16g fat (2g sat. fat), 30mg chol., 640mg sod., 20g carb. (3g sugars, 5g fiber), 23g pro. *Diabetic exchanges:* 3 fat, 2 lean meat, 1 starch, 1 vegetable.

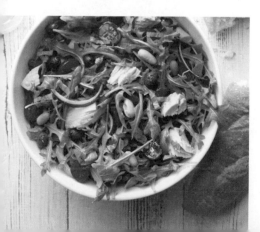

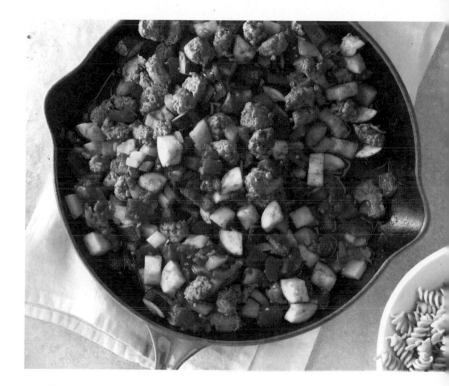

Italian Sausage Veggie Skillet

Serves 6

- 4 cups uncooked whole wheat spiral pasta
- 1 lb. Italian turkey sausage, casings removed
- 1 medium onion, chopped
- 1 garlic clove, minced
- 2 medium zucchini, chopped
- 1 large sweet red pepper, chopped
- 1 large sweet yellow pepper, chopped
- 1 can (28 oz.) diced tomatoes, drained
- ¼ tsp. salt
- ¼ tsp. pepper

- **ONE** Cook pasta according to package directions; drain.
- **TWO** Meanwhile, in large skillet, cook sausage and onion over medium-high heat until sausage is no longer pink, 5-7 minutes. Add garlic and cook 1 minute longer. Add zucchini and peppers; cook until crisp-tender, 3-5 minutes. Add tomatoes, salt and pepper. Cook and stir until vegetables are tender and begin to release their juices, 5-7 minutes. Serve with pasta.

1⅓ cups: 251 cal., 6g fat (1g sat. fat), 28mg chol., 417mg sod., 35g carb. (4g sugars, 6g fiber), 16g pro. *Diabetic exchanges:* 2 vegetable, 2 lean meat, 1½ starch.

Main Meals

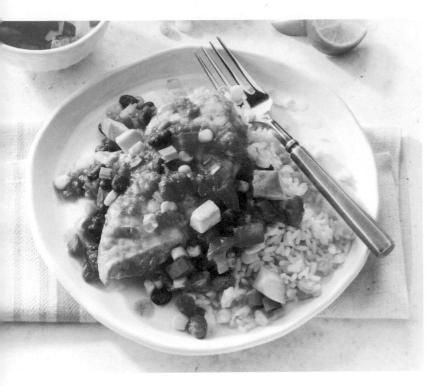

Pepper-Crusted Pork Tenderloin

Serves 6

- 3 Tbsp. Dijon mustard
- 1 Tbsp. buttermilk
- 2 tsp. minced fresh thyme
- 1 to 2 tsp. coarsely ground pepper
- ¼ tsp. salt
- 2 pork tenderloins (¾ lb. each)
- ⅔ cup soft bread crumbs

- **ONE** Preheat oven to 425°. Mix first five ingredients. To make a double roast, arrange tenderloins side by side, thick end to thin end; tie together with kitchen string at 1½-in. intervals. Place on a rack in a 15x10x1-in. pan. Spread with mustard mixture; cover with bread crumbs, pressing to adhere.

- **TWO** Bake until a thermometer inserted in pork reads 145°, 30-40 minutes. (Tent loosely with foil if needed to prevent overbrowning.) Let stand about 5 minutes. Cut into slices; remove string before serving.

1 serving: 155 cal., 4g fat (1g sat. fat), 64mg chol., 353mg sod., 3g carb. (0 sugars, 0 fiber), 23g pro. ***Diabetic exchanges:*** 3 lean meat.

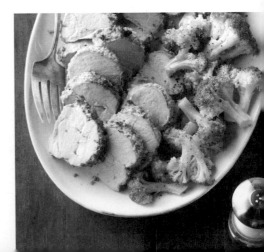

Slow-Cooker Salsa Chicken

Serves 4

- 3 Tbsp. Dijon mustard
- 4 bonelessskinlesschicken breast halves (6 oz. each)
- 1½ cups salsa
- 1 cup frozen corn, thawed
- 1 cup canned no-salt-added pinto beans, rinsed and drained
- 1 cup canned no-salt-added black beans, rinsed and drained
- 1 can (10 oz.) diced tomatoes and green chiles, undrained
- ¼ tsp. pepper

Optional: Hot cooked rice, cubed avocado, chopped fresh tomato, sliced green onions and lime wedges

- **PLACE** chicken in a 4- or 5-qt. slow cooker. Top with salsa, corn, beans, diced tomatoes and chiles and pepper. Cook, covered, on low until a thermometer inserted in chicken reads 165°, 3-4 hours. If desired, serve with optional ingredients.

1 chicken breast half with 1 cup bean mixture: 360 cal., 5g fat (1g sat. fat), 94mg chol., 742mg sod., 35g carb. (5g sugars, 8g fiber), 35g pro. ***Diabetic exchanges:*** 5 lean meat, 2 starch.

Side Dishes

Sweet Potato Kale Pilaf

Serves 8

- 1 cup uncooked wild rice
- 2¼ cups vegetable broth or water
- 1 tsp. olive oil
- 4 bacon strips, chopped
- 1 lb. fresh asparagus, trimmed and cut into 2-in. pieces
- 1 large sweet potato, peeled and chopped
- ½ cup chopped red onion
- 1 cup chopped fresh kale
- 1 garlic clove, minced
- ½ tsp. salt
- ½ tsp. pepper
  Chopped fresh parsley

- **ONE** Rinse wild rice; drain. In a large saucepan, combine broth, rice and oil; bring to a boil. Reduce heat; simmer, covered, until rice is fluffy and tender, 50-55 minutes. Drain.

- **TWO** Meanwhile, in a large skillet, cook bacon over medium heat until crisp. Remove to paper towels to drain. Add asparagus, sweet potato and onion to drippings; cook and stir over medium-high heat until potatoes are crisp-tender, 8-10 minutes.

- **THREE** Stir in kale, garlic, salt and pepper. Cook and stir until vegetables are tender, 8-10 minutes. Stir in rice and reserved bacon. Sprinkle with parsley.

¾ cup: 156 cal., 5g fat (2g sat. fat), 7mg chol., 350mg sod., 23g carb. (5g sugars, 3g fiber), 5g pro. **Diabetic exchanges:** 1½ starch, 1 fat.

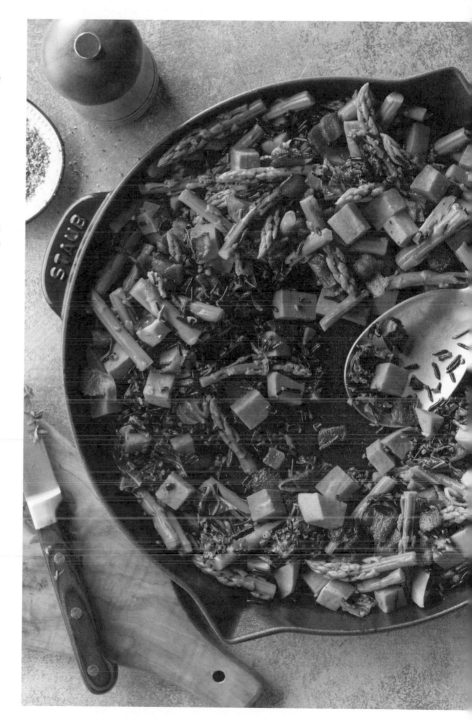

Side Dishes

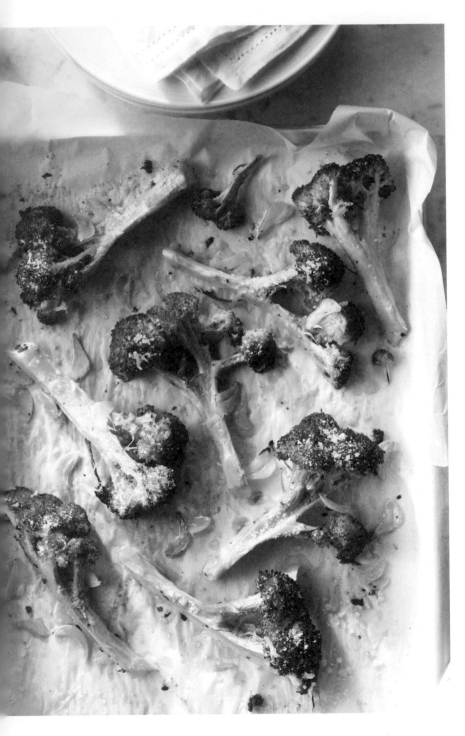

Parmesan Roasted Broccoli

Serves 4

- 2 small broccoli crowns (about 8 oz. each)
- 3 Tbsp. olive oil
- ½ tsp. salt
- ½ tsp. pepper
- ¼ tsp. crushed red pepper flakes
- 4 garlic cloves, thinly sliced
- 2 Tbsp. grated Parmesan cheese
- 1 tsp. grated lemon zest

- **ONE** Preheat oven to 425°. Cut broccoli crowns into quarters from top to bottom. Drizzle with oil; sprinkle with salt, pepper and pepper flakes. Place in a parchment-lined 15x10x1-in. pan.

- **TWO** Roast until crisp-tender, 10-12 minutes. Sprinkle with garlic; roast 5 minutes longer. Sprinkle with cheese; roast until cheese is melted and stalks of broccoli are tender, 2-4 minutes longer. Sprinkle with lemon zest.

2 broccoli pieces: 144 cal., 11g fat (2g sat. fat), 2mg chol., 378mg sod., 9g carb. (2g sugars, 3g fiber), 4g pro. *Diabetic exchanges:* 2 fat, 1 vegetable.

Green Beans in Red Pepper Sauce

Serves 6

- 1 lb. fresh green beans, trimmed
- ½ cup roasted sweet red peppers
- ¼ cup sliced almonds
- 2 Tbsp. olive oil
- 2 Tbsp. minced fresh parsley
- 2 Tbsp. lemon juice
- 2 garlic cloves, halved
- ½ tsp. salt

- **PLACE** beans in a large saucepan; add water to cover. Bring to a boil. Cook, covered, until crisp-tender, 2-4 minutes. Drain. Pulse remaining ingredients in a food processor until smooth. Toss with beans.

¾ cup: 95 cal., 7g fat (1g sat. fat), 0 chol., 276mg sod., 8g carb. (3g sugars, 3g fiber), 2g pro. **Diabetic exchanges:** 1 vegetable, 1 fat.

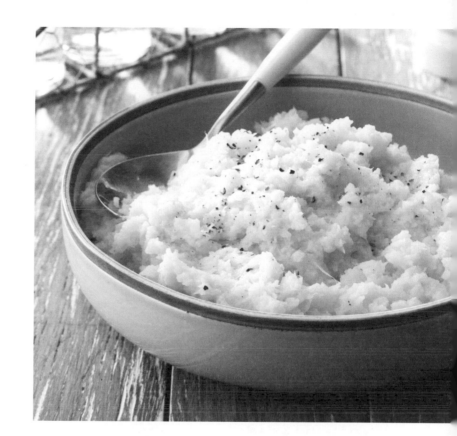

Cauliflower Mash

Serves 6

- 1 large head cauliflower, chopped (about 6 cups)
- ½ cup chicken broth
- 2 garlic cloves, crushed
- 1 tsp. whole peppercorns
- 1 bay leaf
- ½ tsp. salt

- **ONE** Place cauliflower in a large saucepan; add water to cover. Bring to a boil. Reduce heat. Simmer, covered, until tender, 10-12 minutes. Drain; return to pan.

- **TWO** Meanwhile, combine remaining ingredients in a small saucepan. Bring to a boil. Immediately remove from heat and strain; discard garlic, peppercorns and bay leaf. Add broth to cauliflower. Mash to reach desired consistency.

⅔ cup: 26 cal., 0 fat (0 sat. fat), 0 chol., 308mg sod., 5g carb. (2g sugars, 2g fiber), 2g pro. **Diabetic exchanges:** 1 vegetable.

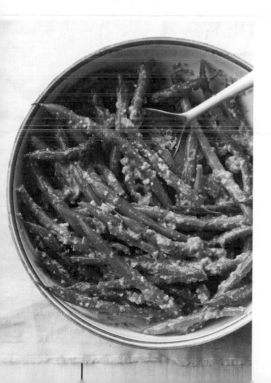

229

Side Dishes

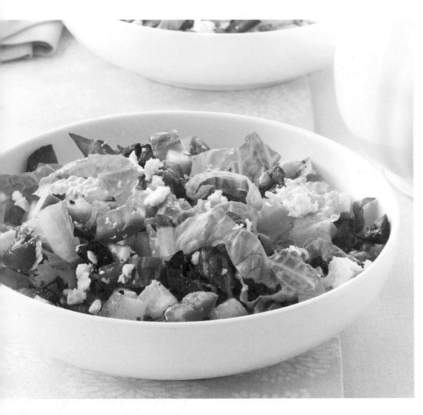

Three-Pepper Coleslaw
Serves 8

- 1 pkg. (10 oz.) angel hair coleslaw mix
- 1 medium sweet red pepper, finely chopped
- 1 medium green pepper, finely chopped
- 1 to 2 jalapeno peppers, seeded and finely chopped
- 3 green onions, chopped
- ¼ cup white wine vinegar
- 2 Tbsp. lime juice
- 2 tsp. canola oil
- 1 tsp. sugar
- ½ tsp. salt
- ¼ tsp. pepper

- **PLACE** the first 5 ingredients in a large serving bowl. In a small bowl, whisk the remaining ingredients. Pour over coleslaw mixture; toss to coat. Cover and refrigerate for at least 30 minutes before serving.

¾ cup: 36 cal., 1g fat (0 sat. fat), 0 chol., 158mg sod., 6g carb. (3g sugars, 2g fiber), 1g pro. **Diabetic exchanges:** 1 vegetable.

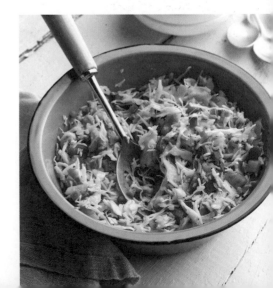

Feta Romaine Salad
Serves 6

- 1 bunch romaine, chopped
- 3 plum tomatoes, seeded and chopped
- 1 cup (4 oz.) crumbled feta cheese
- 1 cup chopped seeded cucumber
- ½ cup Greek olives, chopped
- 2 Tbsp. minced fresh parsley
- 2 Tbsp. minced fresh cilantro
- 3 Tbsp. lemon juice
- 2 Tbsp. olive oil
- ¼ tsp. pepper

- **IN** a large bowl, combine the first seven ingredients. In a small bowl, whisk the remaining ingredients. Drizzle over salad; toss to coat. Serve immediately.

1⅓ cups: 139 cal., 11g fat (3g sat. fat), 10mg chol., 375mg sod., 6g carb. (2g sugars, 3g fiber), 5g pro. **Diabetic exchanges:** 2 fat, 1 vegetable.

Brussels Sprouts with Bacon

Serves 6

3	bacon strips
1¼	lbs. fresh or frozen Brussels sprouts, thawed, quartered
1	large onion, chopped
2	Tbsp. water
¼	tsp. salt
⅛	tsp. pepper
2	Tbsp. balsamic vinegar

● **ONE** In a large skillet, cook bacon over medium heat until crisp. Remove to paper towels; drain, reserving 1 Tbsp. drippings. Crumble bacon and set aside.

● **TWO** In the same pan, saute Brussels sprouts and onion in reserved drippings until crisp-tender. Add the water, salt and pepper. Bring to a boil. Reduce heat; cover and simmer for 4-5 minutes or until Brussels sprouts are tender. Stir in bacon and vinegar.

⅔ cup: 90 cal., 4g fat (1g sat. fat), 6mg chol., 200mg sod., 11g carb. (1g sugars, 4g fiber), 5g pro. ***Diabetic exchanges:*** 1 vegetable, 1 fat.

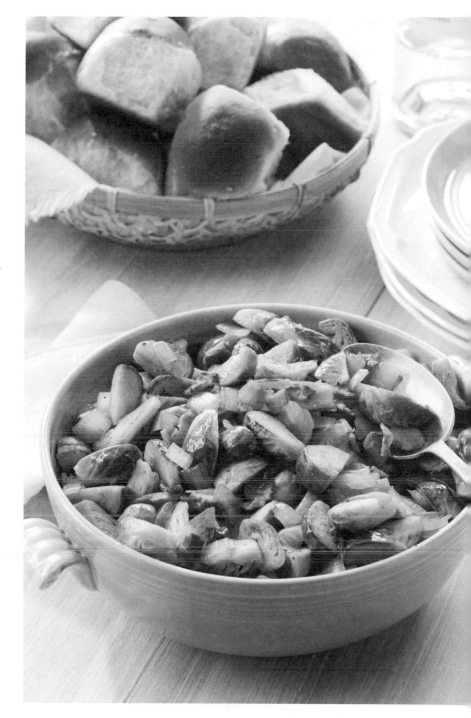

Side Dishes

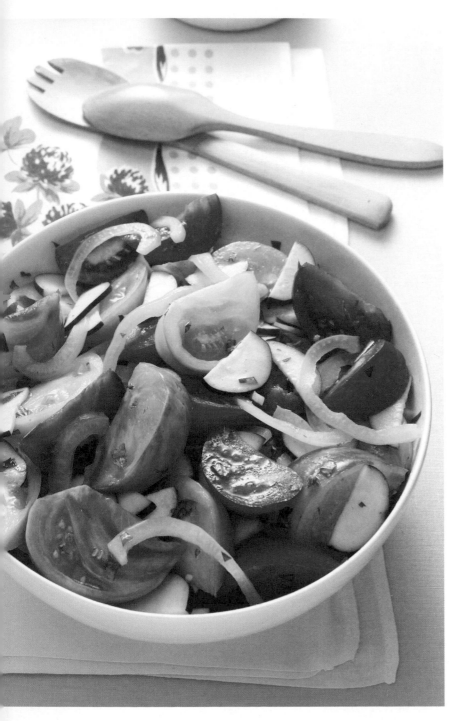

Heirloom Tomato & Zucchini Salad

Serves 12 (1 cup each)

7	large heirloom tomatoes (about 2½ lbs.), cut into wedges
3	medium zucchini, halved lengthwise and thinly sliced
2	medium sweet yellow peppers, thinly sliced
⅓	cup cider vinegar
3	Tbsp. olive oil
1	Tbsp. sugar
1½	tsp. salt
1	Tbsp. each minced fresh basil, parsley and tarragon

● **ONE** In a large bowl, combine tomatoes, zucchini and peppers. In a small bowl, whisk vinegar, oil, sugar and salt until blended. Stir in herbs.

● **TWO** Just before serving, drizzle dressing over salad; toss gently to coat.

1 cup: 68 cal., 4g fat (1g sat. fat), 0 chol., 306mg sod., 8g carb. (5g sugars, 2g fiber), 2g pro. *Diabetic exchanges:* 1 vegetable, ½ fat.

Tabbouleh

Serves 8

- ¼ cup bulgur
- 3 bunches fresh parsley, minced (about 2 cups)
- 3 large tomatoes, finely chopped
- 1 small onion, finely chopped
- ¼ cup lemon juice
- ¼ cup olive oil
- 5 fresh mint leaves, minced
- ½ tsp. salt
- ½ tsp. pepper
- ¼ tsp. cayenne pepper

● **PREPARE** bulgur according to package directions; cool. Transfer to a large bowl. Stir in remaining ingredients. If desired, chill before serving.

⅔ cup: 100 cal., 7g fat (1g sat. fat), 0 chol., 164mg sod., 9g carb. (3g sugars, 2g fiber), 2g pro. **Diabetic exchanges:** 1½ fat, ½ starch.

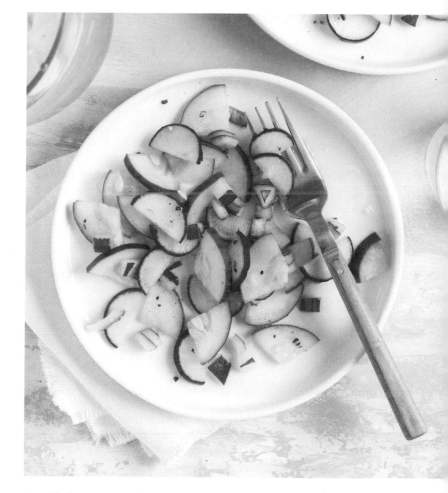

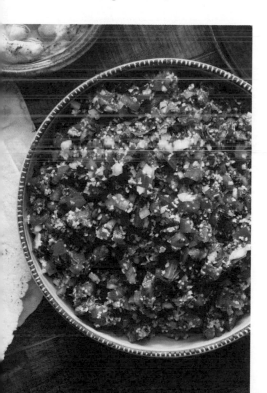

Radish Cucumber Salad

Serves 2

- ½ medium cucumber, halved and sliced
- 2 radishes, sliced
- 2 Tbsp. chopped red onion
- 1 Tbsp. olive oil
- 1½ tsp. lemon juice
- ⅛ to ¼ tsp. garlic salt
- ⅛ tsp. lemon-pepper seasoning

● **IN** a serving bowl, combine the cucumber, radishes and onion. In another bowl, combine the remaining ingredients. Pour over vegetables and toss to coat. Serve immediately.

1 serving: 77 cal., 7g fat (1g sat. fat), 0 chol., 143mg sod., 4g carb. (2g sugars, 1g fiber), 1g pro. **Diabetic exchanges:** 1½ fat, 1 vegetable.

233

Snacks

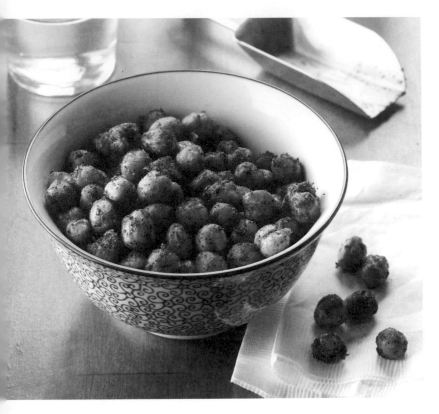

Gorgonzola Tomatoes on Endive

Makes 20 appetizers

- 20 leaves Belgian endive (about 2 heads)
- 2 medium tomatoes, seeded and finely chopped
- 3 green onions, thinly sliced
- ½ cup crumbled Gorgonzola cheese
- ½ cup chopped walnuts, toasted
- ⅓ cup balsamic vinaigrette

● **ARRANGE** endive on a serving platter. In each leaf, layer the tomatoes, green onions, cheese and walnuts. Drizzle with vinaigrette. Chill until serving.

1 appetizer: 49 cal., 4g fat (1g sat. fat), 3mg chol., 84mg sod., 4g carb. (1g sugars, 2g fiber), 2g pro. ***Diabetic exchanges:*** 1 fat.

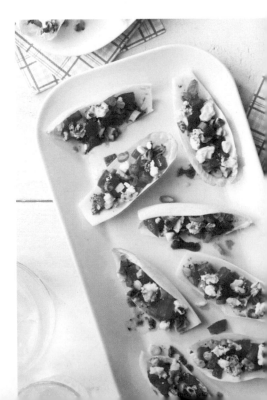

Chili-Lime Roasted Chickpeas

Makes 2 cups

- 2 cans (15 oz. each) chickpeas or garbanzo beans, rinsed, drained and patted dry
- 2 Tbsp. extra virgin olive oil
- 1 Tbsp. chili powder
- 2 tsp. ground cumin
- 1 tsp. grated lime zest
- 1 Tbsp. lime juice
- ¾ tsp. sea salt

● **ONE** Preheat oven to 400°. Line a 15x10x1-in. baking sheet with foil. Spread chickpeas in a single layer over foil, removing any loose skins. Bake until very crunchy, 40-45 minutes, stirring every 15 minutes.

● **TWO** Meanwhile, whisk together remaining ingredients. Remove chickpeas from oven; let cool 5 minutes. Drizzle with oil mixture; shake pan to coat. Cool completely. Store in an airtight container.

⅓ cup: 178 cal., 8g fat (1g sat. fat), 0 chol., 463mg sod., 23g carb. (3g sugars, 6g fiber), 6g pro. ***Diabetic exchanges:*** 1½ starch, 1½ fat.

Healthy Greek Bean Dip

Makes 3 cups

- 2 cans (15 oz. each) cannellini beans, rinsed and drained
- ¼ cup water
- ¼ cup finely chopped roasted sweet red peppers
- 2 Tbsp. finely chopped red onion
- 2 Tbsp. olive oil
- 2 Tbsp. lemon juice
- 1 Tbsp. snipped fresh dill
- 2 garlic cloves, minced
- ¼ tsp. salt
- ¼ tsp. pepper
- 1 small cucumber, peeled, seeded and finely chopped
- ½ cup fat-free plain Greek yogurt

  Additional snipped fresh dill

  Baked pita chips or assorted fresh vegetables

- **PROCESS** beans and water in a food processor until smooth. Transfer to a greased 1½-qt. slow cooker. Add the next 8 ingredients. Cook, covered, on low until heated through, 2-3 hours. Stir in cucumber and yogurt; cool slightly. Sprinkle with additional dill. Serve warm or cold with chips or assorted fresh vegetables.

¼ cup: 86 cal., 3g fat (0 sat. fat), 0 chol., 260mg sod., 11g carb. (1g sugars, 3g fiber), 4g pro. **Diabetic exchanges:** 1 starch, ½ fat.

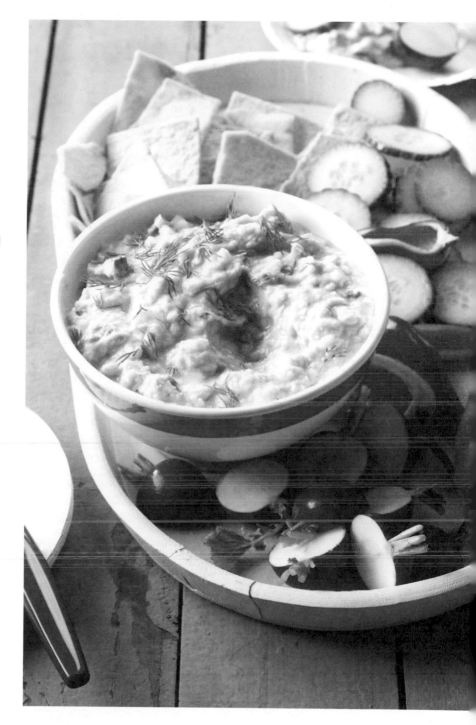

Snacks

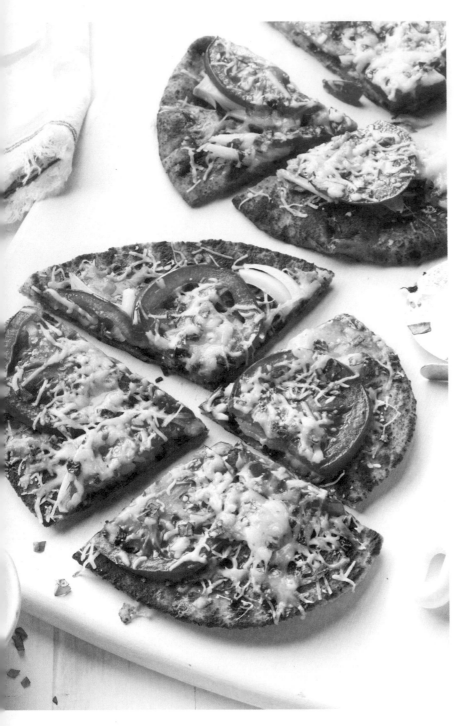

Grilled Garden Veggie Flatbreads

Serves 8

- 2 whole grain naan flatbreads
- 2 tsp. olive oil
- 1 medium yellow or red tomato, thinly sliced
- ¼ cup thinly sliced onion
- ½ cup shredded part-skim mozzarella cheese
- 2 Tbsp. shredded Parmesan cheese
- 1 Tbsp. minced fresh basil
- ½ tsp. garlic powder
- 1 tsp. balsamic vinegar
- ½ tsp. coarse sea salt

- **ONE** Grill flatbreads, covered, over indirect medium heat 2-3 minutes or until bottoms are lightly browned.

- **TWO** Remove from grill. Brush grilled sides with oil; top with tomato and onion to within ½ in. of edges. In a small bowl, toss cheeses with basil and garlic powder; sprinkle over vegetables. Drizzle with vinegar; sprinkle with salt. Return to grill; cook, covered, 2-3 minutes longer or until cheese is melted. Cut into wedges.

1 wedge: 132 cal., 5g fat (2g sat. fat), 8mg chol., 390mg sod., 16g carb. (2g sugars, 2g fiber), 5g pro. **Diabetic exchanges:** 1 starch, 1 fat.

Rosemary Walnuts

Makes 2 cups

- 2 cups walnut halves
  Cooking spray
- 2 tsp. dried rosemary, crushed
- ½ tsp. kosher salt
- ¼ to ½ tsp. cayenne pepper

● **ONE** Place walnuts in a small bowl. Spritz with cooking spray. Add the seasonings; toss to coat. Place in a single layer on a baking sheet.

● **TWO** Bake at 350° for 10 minutes. Serve warm, or cool completely and store in an airtight container.

¼ cup: 166 cal., 17g fat (2g sat. fat), 0 chol., 118mg sod., 4g carb. (1g sugars, 2g fiber), 4g pro. *Diabetic exchanges:* 3 fat.

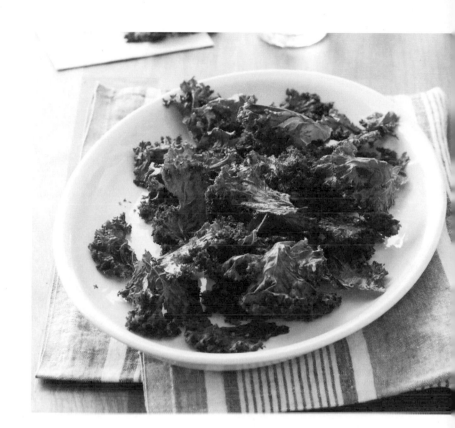

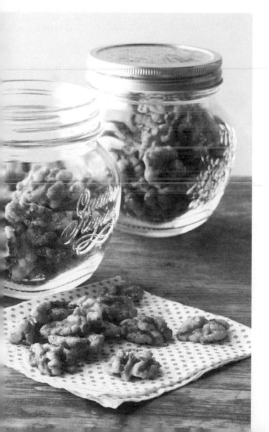

Old Bay Crispy Kale Chips

Serves 4

- 1 bunch kale, washed
- 2 Tbsp. olive oil
- 1 to 3 tsp. Old Bay Seasoning
  Sea salt, to taste

● **ONE** Preheat oven to 300°. Remove tough stems from kale and tear leaves into large pieces. Place in a large bowl. Toss with olive oil and seasonings. Arrange leaves in a single layer on greased baking sheets.

● **TWO** Bake, uncovered, 10 minutes and then rotate pans. Continue baking until crisp and just starting to brown, about 15 minutes longer. Let stand at least 5 minutes before serving.

1 serving: 101 cal., 7g fat (1g sat. fat), 0 chol., 202mg sod., 8g carb. (0 sugars, 2g fiber), 3g pro. *Diabetic exchanges:* 1½ fat, 1 vegetable.

237

Desserts

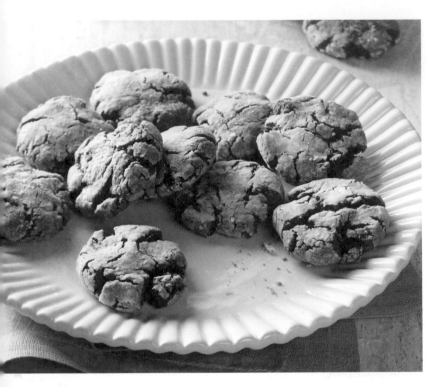

Chunky Banana Cream Freeze

Makes 3 cups

5	medium bananas, peeled and frozen
⅓	cup almond milk
2	Tbsp. unsweetened finely shredded coconut
2	Tbsp. creamy peanut butter
1	tsp. vanilla extract
¼	cup chopped walnuts
3	Tbsp. raisins

- **ONE** Place the bananas, milk, coconut, peanut butter and vanilla in a food processor; cover and process until blended.

- **TWO** Transfer to a freezer container; stir in walnuts and raisins. Freeze for 2-4 hours before serving.

½ cup: 181 cal., 7g fat (2g sat. fat), 0 chol., 35mg sod., 29g carb. (16g sugars, 4g fiber), 3g pro. *Diabetic exchanges:* 1 fruit, 1 fat, ½ starch.

Molasses Crackle Cookies

Makes 2½ dozen

⅔	cup sugar
¼	cup canola oil
1	large egg
⅓	cup molasses
2	cups white whole wheat flour
1½	tsp. baking soda
1	tsp. ground cinnamon
½	tsp. salt
¼	tsp. ground ginger
¼	tsp. ground cloves
1	Tbsp. confectioners' sugar

- **ONE** In a small bowl, beat sugar and oil until blended. Beat in egg and molasses. Combine the flour, baking soda, cinnamon, salt, ginger and cloves; gradually add to sugar mixture and mix well. Cover and refrigerate at least 2 hours.

- **TWO** Preheat oven to 350°. Shape dough into 1-in. balls; roll in confectioners' sugar. Place 2 in. apart on baking sheets coated with cooking spray; flatten slightly. Bake 7-9 minutes or until set. Remove to wire racks to cool.

1 cookie: 77 cal., 2g fat (0 sat. fat), 7mg chol., 106mg sod., 14g carb. (7g sugars, 1g fiber), 1g pro. *Diabetic exchanges:* 1 starch.

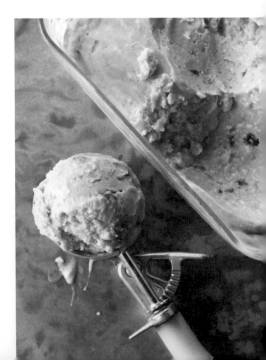

Orange Ricotta Cake Roll

Serves 12

- 4 large eggs, separated, room temperature
- ¼ cup baking cocoa
- 2 Tbsp. all-purpose flour
- ⅛ tsp. salt
- ⅔ cup confectioners' sugar, sifted, divided
- 1 tsp. vanilla extract
- ½ tsp. cream of tartar

Filling

- 1 container (15 oz.) ricotta cheese
- 3 Tbsp. mascarpone cheese
- ⅓ cup sugar
- 1 Tbsp. Kahlua (coffee liqueur)
- 1 Tbsp. grated orange zest
- ½ tsp. vanilla extract
  Additional confectioners' sugar

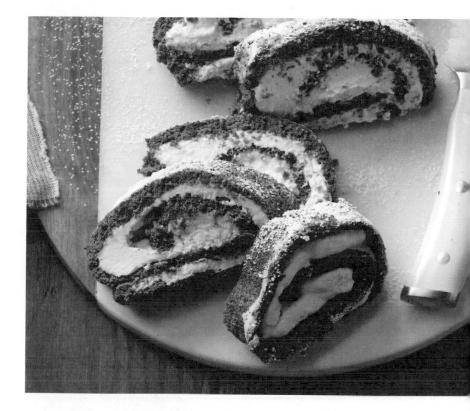

- **ONE** Place egg whites in a bowl. Preheat oven to 325°. Line bottom of a greased 15x10x1-in. baking pan with parchment; grease paper. Sift cocoa, flour and salt together twice.

- **TWO** In a large bowl, beat egg yolks until slightly thickened. Gradually add ⅓ cup confectioners' sugar, beating on high speed until thick and lemon-colored. Beat in vanilla. Fold in cocoa mixture (batter will be very thick).

- **THREE** Add cream of tartar to egg whites; with clean beaters, beat on medium until soft peaks form. Gradually add remaining confectioners' sugar, 1 Tbsp. at a time, beating on high after each addition until sugar is dissolved. Continue beating until soft glossy peaks form. Fold a fourth of the whites into batter, then fold in remaining whites. Transfer to prepared pan, spreading evenly.

- **FOUR** Bake until top springs back when lightly touched, 9-11 minutes. Cover cake with waxed paper; cool completely on a wire rack.

- **FIVE** Remove waxed paper; invert cake onto an 18-in.-long sheet of waxed paper dusted with confectioners' sugar. Gently peel off parchment.

- **SIX** In a small bowl, beat cheeses and sugar until blended. Stir in Kahlua, orange zest and vanilla. Spread over cake to within ½ in. of edges. Roll up jelly-roll style, starting with a short side. Trim ends; place on a platter, seam side down.

- **SEVEN** Refrigerate, covered, at least 1 hour before serving. To serve, dust with confectioners' sugar.

1 slice: 169 cal., 9g fat (5g sat. fat), 94mg chol., 95mg sod., 17g carb. (14g sugars, 0 fiber), 7g pro. *Diabetic exchanges:* 2 fat, 1 starch.

239

Desserts

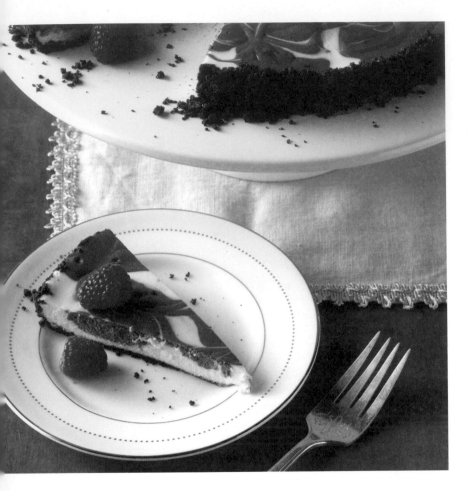

Chocolate Swirled Cheesecake

Serves 12

- 2 cups 2% cottage cheese
- 1 cup crushed chocolate wafers (about 16 wafers)
- 1 pkg. (8 oz.) reduced-fat cream cheese, cubed
- ½ cup sugar
  Dash salt
- 1 Tbsp. vanilla extract
- 2 large eggs, lightly beaten
- 1 large egg white
- 2 oz. bittersweet chocolate, melted and cooled
  Fresh raspberries, optional

ONE Line a strainer with four layers of cheesecloth or one coffee filter; place over a bowl. Place cottage cheese in strainer; refrigerate, covered, 1 hour. Place a 9-in. springform pan on a double thickness of heavy-duty foil (about 18 in. square); wrap foil securely around pan. Coat inside of pan with cooking spray. Press crushed wafers onto bottom and 1 in. up sides.

TWO Preheat oven to 350°. In a food processor, process drained cottage cheese until smooth. Add cream cheese, sugar and salt; process until blended. Transfer to a bowl; stir in vanilla, eggs and egg white. Remove 1 cup batter to a small bowl; stir in melted chocolate.

THREE Pour plain batter into crust. Drop chocolate batter by spoonfuls over plain batter. Cut through batter with a knife to swirl. Place springform pan in a larger baking pan; add 1 in. of boiling water to larger pan.

FOUR Bake until center is just set and top appears dull, about 40 minutes. Turn off oven; open door slightly. Cool cheesecake in oven 30 minutes.

FIVE Remove springform pan from water bath; remove foil. Loosen sides of cheesecake with a knife; cool on a wire rack 30 minutes. Refrigerate overnight, covering when completely cooled.

SIX Remove rim from pan. If desired, top with raspberries.

1 piece: 187 cal., 8g fat (5g sat. fat), 46mg chol., 378mg sod., 17g carb. (14g sugars, 1g fiber), 8g pro. **Diabetic exchanges:** 1½ starch, 1 lean meat, ½ fat.

Cranberry Stuffed Apples

Serves 5

- 5 medium apples
- ⅓ cup fresh or frozen cranberries, thawed and chopped
- ¼ cup packed brown sugar
- 2 Tbsp. chopped walnuts
- ¼ tsp. ground cinnamon
- ⅛ tsp. ground nutmeg
  Optional: Whipped cream or vanilla ice cream

- **ONE** Core apples, leaving bottoms intact. Peel top third of each apple; place in a 5-qt. slow cooker. Combine the cranberries, brown sugar, walnuts, cinnamon and nutmeg; spoon into apples.

- **TWO** Cover and cook on low for 3-4 hours or until apples are tender. Serve with whipped cream or ice cream if desired.

1 stuffed apple: 136 cal., 2g fat (0 sat. fat), 0 chol., 6mg sod., 31g carb. (25g sugars, 4g fiber), 1g pro. **Diabetic exchanges:** 1 starch, 1 fruit.

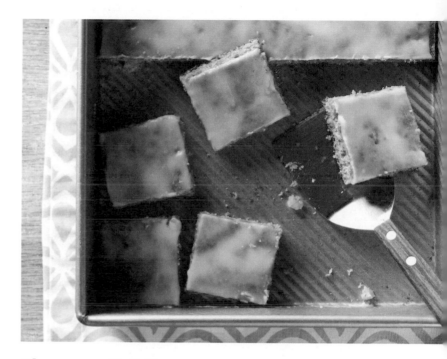

Cinnamon Nut Bars

Makes 2 dozen

- ½ cup whole wheat flour
- ½ cup all-purpose flour
- ½ cup sugar
- 1½ tsp. ground cinnamon
- 1¼ tsp. baking powder
- ¼ tsp. baking soda
- 1 large egg, room temperature, beaten
- ⅓ cup canola oil
- ¼ cup unsweetened applesauce
- ¼ cup honey
- 1 cup chopped walnuts

Icing

- 1 cup confectioners' sugar
- 2 Tbsp. butter, melted
- 1 tsp. vanilla extract
- 1 Tbsp. water
- 2 Tbsp. honey

- **ONE** Preheat oven to 350°. In a large bowl, combine flours, sugar, cinnamon, baking powder and baking soda. In another bowl, combine egg, oil, applesauce and honey. Stir into dry ingredients just until moistened. Fold in walnuts.

- **TWO** Spread batter into a 13x9-in. baking pan coated with cooking spray. Bake 15-20 minutes or until a toothpick inserted in the center comes out clean.

- **THREE** Combine icing ingredients; spread over warm bars. Cool completely before cutting into bars.

1 bar: 142 cal., 7g fat (1g sat. fat), 11mg chol., 44mg sod., 18g carb. (13g sugars, 1g fiber), 2g pro. **Diabetic exchanges:** 1 starch, 1 fat.

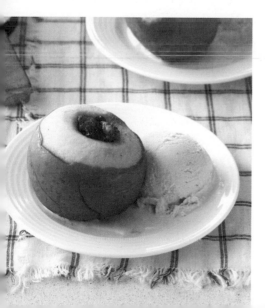

Desserts

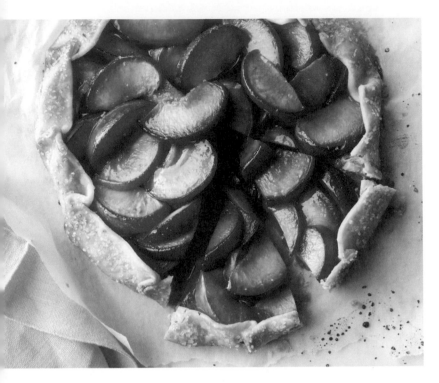

Ginger Plum Tart

Serves 8

- 1 sheet refrigerated pie crust
- 3½ cups sliced fresh plums (about 10 medium)
- 3 Tbsp. plus 1 tsp. coarse sugar, divided
- 1 Tbsp. cornstarch
- 2 tsp. finely chopped crystallized ginger
- 1 large egg white
- 1 Tbsp. water

- **ONE** Preheat oven to 400°. On a work surface, unroll crust. Roll to a 12-in. circle. Transfer to a parchment-lined baking sheet.

- **TWO** In a large bowl, toss plums with 3 Tbsp. sugar and cornstarch. Arrange plums on crust to within 2 in. of edges; sprinkle with ginger. Fold crust edge over plums, pleating as you go.

- **THREE** In a small bowl, whisk egg white and water; brush over folded crust. Sprinkle with remaining sugar.

- **FOUR** Bake until crust is golden brown, 20-25 minutes. Cool in pan on a wire rack. Serve warm or at room temperature.

1 piece: 190 cal., 7g fat (3g sat. fat), 5mg chol., 108mg sod., 30g carb. (14g sugars, 1g fiber), 2g pro. *Diabetic exchanges:* 1½ starch, 1 fat, ½ fruit.

Light & Creamy Chocolate Pudding

Serves 4

- 3 Tbsp. cornstarch
- 2 Tbsp. sugar
- 2 Tbsp. baking cocoa
- ⅛ tsp. salt
- 2 cups chocolate soy milk
- 1 tsp. vanilla extract

- **ONE** In a small heavy saucepan, mix cornstarch, sugar, cocoa and salt. Whisk in milk. Cook and stir over medium heat until thickened and bubbly. Reduce heat to low; cook and stir 2 minutes longer.

- **TWO** Remove from heat. Stir in vanilla. Cool 15 minutes, stirring occasionally.

- **THREE** Transfer to dessert dishes. Refrigerate, covered, 30 minutes or until cold.

½ cup: 127 cal., 2g fat (0 sat. fat), 0 chol., 112mg sod., 25g carb. (16g sugars, 1g fiber), 3g pro. *Diabetic exchanges:* 1½ starch.

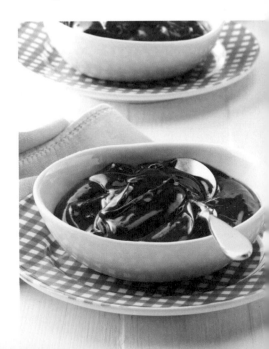

Sample Meal Plans

DAY 1

Breakfast
1 piece *Colorful Pepper Frittata* (p. 201), 2 slices whole wheat toast, 2 tsp. butter, 2 clementines

Snack
6 ounces no-sugar-added Greek yogurt, 1 medium apple

Lunch
1 serving *Herbed Tuna & White Bean Salad* (p. 225), 2 whole grain crispy breadsticks, 1 cup fat-free milk

Snack
½ cup *Chunky Banana Cream Freeze* (p. 238)

Dinner
1 serving *Chicken Thighs with Shallots & Spinach* (p. 214), ¾ cup *Green Beans in Red Pepper Sauce* (p. 229), ½ cup brown rice, 1 cup fat-free milk

Snack
¼ cup *Healthy Greek Bean Dip* (p. 235) + 1 cup nonstarchy veggies

DAY 2

Breakfast
1 serving *Pear Quinoa Breakfast Bake* (p. 198), ½ cup raspberries

Snack
¼ cup *Healthy Greek Bean Dip* (p. 235) + 1 cup nonstarchy veggies, 1 string cheese

Lunch
1¼ cups *Italian Sausage Zucchini Soup* (p. 210), 1 wedge *Grilled Garden Veggie Flatbreads* (p. 236), ½ cup 2% cottage cheese

Snack
6 oz. no-sugar-added Greek yogurt, 1 small banana

Dinner
1 *Fiery Stuffed Poblano* (p. 219), 1 serving *Radish Cucumber Salad* (p. 233), 1 cup fat-free milk

Snack
1 *Cranberry Stuffed Apple* (p. 241), 1 cup fat-free milk

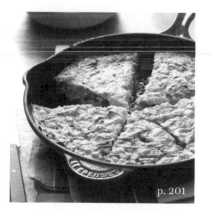
p. 201

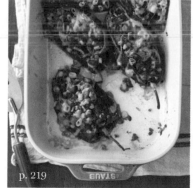
p. 219

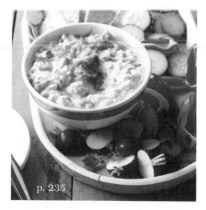
p. 235

Sample Meal Plans

| DAY 3 | GENERIC DAY 1 |

Breakfast
1 serving *Poached Eggs with Tarragon Asparagus* (p. 204), ¾ cup cubed fresh pineapple, 1 cup fat-free milk

Snack
6 oz. no-sugar-added Greek yogurt

Lunch
1 *Tomato & Avocado Sandwich* (p. 205), 1⅓ cups *Feta Romaine Salad* (p. 230), 1 medium apple

Snack
1 *Cinnamon Nut Bar* (p. 241), 1 cup fat-free milk

Dinner
1 *Lemony Grilled Salmon Fillet with Dill Sauce* (p. 212), 1 small baked potato, 1 cup *Heirloom Tomato & Zucchini Salad* (p. 232)

Snack
⅓ cup *Chili-Lime Roasted Chickpeas* (p. 234), ¾ cup sliced strawberries

Breakfast
1 cup cooked oatmeal, 6 oz. no-sugar-added soy milk yogurt

Snack
2 Tbsp. hummus with 1 cup nonstarchy veggies, 1 cup plain unsweetened soy milk

Lunch
1½ cups lentil vegetable soup, 2 whole grain crackers, ¾ cup red grapes

Snack
¼ cup walnuts, ¾ cup sliced fresh strawberries

Dinner
1 small sweet potato with ½ cup black beans and ¼ cup salsa, 2 cups salad greens with 2 Tbsp. vinaigrette, 1 cup plain unsweetened soy milk

Snack
1 medium apple with 2 Tbsp. almond butter

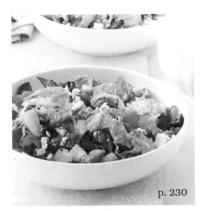

p. 230

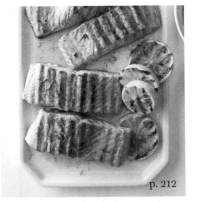

p. 212

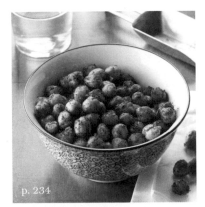

p. 234

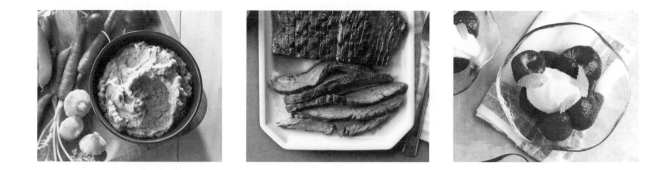

GENERIC DAY 2

Breakfast
1 cup Wheaties, 1 cup fat-free milk, 1 small banana,
1 slice whole wheat toast, 1 tsp. butter

Snack
¼ cup almonds, 1 medium apple

Lunch
3 oz. cooked skinless chicken breast on 2 cups salad
greens with ¼ cup croutons and 2 Tbsp. vinaigrette,
1 whole wheat dinner roll, 1 cup fat-free milk

Snack
6 oz. no-sugar-added Greek yogurt

Dinner
3 oz. cooked flank steak, 1½ cups sauteed
zucchini with cherry tomatoes, ½ cup cooked
whole wheat orzo, hot tea or water

Snack
¾ cup sliced fresh strawberries with
2 Tbsp. whipped cream

GENERIC DAY 3

Breakfast
2 small whole wheat pancakes, 1 tsp. butter,
1 Tbsp. maple syrup, ½ cup raspberries,
1 scrambled egg, 1 cup fat-free milk

Snack
2 Tbsp. hummus with 1 cup nonstarchy veggies

Lunch
1 turkey sandwich (2 oz. cooked turkey, lettuce,
tomato, red onion, 1 Tbsp. mayonnaise, 2 slices
whole wheat bread), 2 cups salad greens with
2 Tbsp. vinaigrette, 1 cup fat-free milk

Snack
¾ cup red grapes, 1 oz. cheese, ¼ cup walnut halves

Dinner
3 oz. cooked pork loin chop, ¾ cup roasted
potato cubes, 1½ cups roasted asparagus with
summer squash, hot tea or water

Snack
½ whole wheat English muffin with 1 Tbsp.
no-sugar-added peanut butter, 1 cup fat-free milk

Index